Endorsements

"As someone interested and engaged in advancing value-based procurement approaches in healthcare, I see this book as a timely and practical resource. It captures the essence of innovation procurement: turning procurement from a transactional exercise into a strategic driver of healthcare transformation. The insights gathered by the Procure4Health partners, under the editorship of Professor Hamish Laing, will inspire and empower procurers across Europe to embrace innovation and deliver value for patients and health systems."

Hans Bax, Digital Health and MedTech Value, Senior Advisor Value & Innovation-Based Access, MedTech Europe

"This book represents the work of those with similar concerns who seek to make public procurement the tool that has a direct impact on the improvement of healthcare processes and, ultimately, on the improvement of citizens' health. It is a must read for all procurement professionals, innovative industry, managers, academics, clinicians and policy makers who work for and with public health systems."

Susana Alvarez, ARGES Health and Society, Former Deputy Director General of Public Procurement for the Madrid Health Service

"Healthcare in Europe faces the dual challenge of sustainability and innovation. This book captures the spirit of the Procure4Health initiative in showing how procurement, when used strategically, can bridge the gap between innovation and implementation. It is an essential read for those committed to shaping the future of health systems through collaboration and smarter investment."

Michele Calabrò, Executive Director of the European Regional and Local Health Authorities (EUREGHA) and Co-Chair of the European Alliance for Value in Health (EAVH).

"Drawing on insights from Procure4Health and other leading EU initiatives, this guide introduces readers to the opportunities and expectations of modern procurement processes. Whether preparing for tenders, facilitating market participation, or driving sustainable procurement outcomes, this book provides relevant resources needed to contribute to the transformation of healthcare."

Rossana Alessandrello is Value Based Procurement Coordinator at AQuAS – Agència de Qualitat i Avaluació Sanitàries de Catalunya. She also serves as Coordinator of the Value Based Procurement Subcommission of the Innovation & Transformation Departmental Commission of the Catalonian Health System

IMPLEMENTING INNOVATION PROCUREMENT IN HEALTHCARE

IMPLEMENTING INNOVATION PROCUREMENT IN HEALTHCARE

From Vision to Value

Procure4Health

Hamish Laing

Published by Sea Pen Books 2025

Sea Pen Books Ltd
18 Northburn Avenue
Rubislaw
Aberdeen
Aberdeenshire
Scotland
United Kingdom
AB15 6AH

www.seapenbooks.com

A CIP catalogue record for this book is available from the British Library

ISBN: 978-1-0683764-7-4

Printed and Bound in Great Britain by CPI Antony Rowe
Bumpers Farm Industrial Estate
Chippenham
Wiltshire
SN14 6LH

Typeset by Deanta, 8 The Seapoint Building, 44-45 Clontarf Road, Clontarf, Dublin 3, Ireland

Contents

Acknowledgements

We would like to thank all the founding partners of the Procure4Health project who have participated in the Work Packages, General Assembly meetings, Twinning Events and many other activities during the lifetime of the project that have shaped the content of this book.

Particular thanks go to the project technical team from SAS, FPS, ZENIT, RESAH, SHI, HCWH, CORVERS, TICBIOMED, ISAB, EMPIRICA, SILO and ZOZ SB for the co-ordination and energy that they have brought to a complex multi-stakeholder and multinational project. They have also disseminated the learning that has resulted to a much wider group of stakeholders who have been affiliated to this project. None of this would have been possible without the exceptional leadership of Carlos Larrañeta Gómez-Caminero, Procure4Health's project co-ordinator. A special mention for Karsten Lemke, one of our exceptional contributors, who sadly passed away just after this book was completed. Our condolences to his family and friends.

This book represents a further stage in knowledge dissemination as the project concludes; sharing the learning widely with the public health procurement community, healthcare provider organisations, industry suppliers and anyone interested in the development and procurement of innovation for use in healthcare. It brings together a series of essays that were published as "insights" on the project website during the lifetime of the Procure4Health project. We thank the authors for their permission to create a publicly available compendium of their work through this book.

We are very grateful to Julia Swales, our publisher, for her advice, support and tolerance of our timelines and requirements, and to Nikki Bramhill for her suggestions. Thanks also to Lola Salinas for her help with the book design and content co-ordination.

Procure4Health was funded through the Horizon EU programme, and we thank the EU Commission for recognising the importance of the project and investing in it. We believe that we have realised considerable value from that investment through all the project deliverables and the strong networks of procurers from across Europe that we have created to share knowledge, and which will endure.

Hamish Laing
Editor

Procure4Health Founding Partner Organisations

SERVICIO ANDALUZ DE SALUD (SAS)	Spain
ZENIT GmbH	Germany
RESEAU DES ACHETEURS HOSPITALIERS IDF (GIP RESAH)	France
SYKEHUSINNKJØP HF	Norway
CORVERS PROCUREMENT SERVICES BV	Spain
TICBIOMED	Spain
HEALTHCARE WITHOUT HARM EUROPE (HCWH EUROPE)	Belgium
INNOVATION SKÅNE AB (ISAB)	Sweden
EMPIRICA	Germany
SCIENCE & INNOVATION LINK OFFICE (SILO)	Spain
ZOZ SUCHA BESKIDZKA (ZOZ SB)	Poland
MINISTRY OF HEALTH, REPUBLIC OF TÜRKIYE	Türkiye
SERVIZO GALEGO DE SAÚDE	Spain
SERVICOS PARTILHADOS DA MINISTÉRIO DE SAÚDE	Portugal
WOJEWÓDZKI SZPITAL SPECJALISTYCZNY W OLSZTYNIE	Poland
AZIENDA REGIONALE PER L'INNOVAZIONE E GLI ACQUISTI (ARIA)	Italy
SERVICIO ARAGONES DE SALUD	Spain
REGIONAAL HAIGLA	Estonia
UNIVERSITY OF THESSALY	Greece
REGION VÄSTERBOTTEN	Sweden
ATRYS PORTUGAL CENTRO MEDICO AVANCADO	Portugal
REGION HOVEDSTADEN	Denmark
MERCURHOSP	Belgium
NATIONAL SERVICES SCOTLAND	UK
NHS WALES SHARED SERVICES PROCUREMENT	UK
SWANSEA UNIVERSITY	UK

Full details of Procure4Health may be found at: https://procure4health.eu/

About the Authors

Carlos Larrañeta Gómez-Caminero was the Coordinator of the Procure4Health project and is the Head of the Public Procurement of Innovation Technical Office within the Andalusian Public Health System (APHS), responsible for the provision of healthcare to the population of Andalusia (8.6 million inhabitants). The office, part of the Progress and Health Foundation (FPS), gives support to the Andalusian Public Procurement for Innovation in Health Programme, manages the configuration of the Early Demand Map of the APHS and promotes and manages PPI projects in health in Andalusia.

Björn Lagnevik is an Innovation Procurement Design Strategist at Innovation Skåne AB, an innovation company fully owned by Region Skåne, the County Council of the southernmost county in Sweden, which has approximately 1.4 million inhabitants. Region Skåne is responsible for the public healthcare system and regional economic development, including innovation and growth, regional infrastructure, digitalisation, culture and public transportation. As a regional innovation company, Innovation Skåne, together with private and public actors, guides and develops new opportunities for innovation and growth that improve Skåne, as well as the world.

Diana Cortés Rodríguez is a Senior Consultant in Business Process Services of the Public Unit and Senior Research & Development Consultant at SILO, a management consulting firm, with headquarters in Madrid. SILO is a knowledge-intensive, policy-oriented small- and medium-sized enterprises (SMEs) specialist in science and innovation governance, Innovation Procurement, and knowledge and technology circulation in the international context. SILO has unique knowledge of the health and biotechnology sector that allows the company to work with hospitals, administrations and innovative companies in the biotechnology, pharmaceutical and health technology sectors. SILO has collaborated with the main Health Services and Departments at a national level to assist them in the implementation of Public Procurement of Innovation projects.

Jorge González is the Director of Ticbiomed Spain, an association specialising in Digital Health whose mission is to drive the digital transformation of European healthcare. Their main goal is to add value to their partners, creating synergies at a national and European level while connecting opportunities with innovative solutions in Digital Health. Ticbiomed helps healthcare organisations and regional healthcare providers identify their innovation challenges, in accordance with their global strategy, with the goal that the offer gets adapted to their needs. Ticbiomed supports the leadership of innovative healthcare professionals and encourages open innovation from the demand-side.

Ana Lucia Jaramillo Villacís (Legal Procurement Researcher), **Beatriz Gómez Fariñas** (Legal Procurement Consultant) and **Azra Atalan** (Legal Procurement Consultant) are part of the legal team at Corvers in Spain and have experience in Innovation Procurement projects across Europe and beyond. Corvers has extensive experience in helping public buyers take advantage of the many benefits of using Innovation Procurement and to leverage their procurement plans to the next level.

Nazan Aynur is a Medical Technology Consultant and **Karsten Lemke** was a Project Manager and Innovation Consultant at ZENIT GmbH, the innovation and European agency of the state of North Rhine-Westphalia (NRW). On behalf of the EU, federal and state governments, ZENIT provides services for companies, especially small- and medium-sized enterprises, as well as for universities and research institutions within NRW, the rest of Germany and abroad. ZENIT supports SMEs and researchers in all their innovation activities, from the search for suitable funding programmes for innovations to the search for suitable cooperation partners for research and development projects and the creation of market entry strategies abroad. Within the Procure4Health project, ZENIT was responsible for the Market Analysis and the related Open Market Consultations (OMCs).

Klaus Piesche, Sonja Müller and Lutz Kubitschke are Senior Consultants at Empirica Technology and Communication Research based in Bonn, Germany. Empirica specialises in research and consultancy in the fields of healthcare, ITC, energy and innovation, bridging the gap between policy, technology, and practical application. Over the last eight years, empirica has been involved in numerous Pre-Commercial Procurements in the areas of health and care (and energy), covering pretty much all aspects that benefit from non-procurer support: from requirements engineering to drafting tender documents, organising Open Market Consultations, and providing support during evaluations and throughout the three phases.

Ali Fakih is a Sustainable Innovation Officer, Healthcare Without Harm (HCWH), a not-for-profit member-based organisation that exists to create a sustainable healthcare sector: one that does no harm to patients and our planet. HCWH inspires action across society to protect human and environmental health and drive change in communities for people to live more healthily on a healthier planet. Members across Europe include healthcare professionals and organisations, healthcare systems, local and regional authorities, academics and more, transforming how healthcare systems work.

Hamish Laing is a Professor of Enhanced Innovation, Engagement and Outcomes and the Director of the Value-Based Health and Care Academy in the School of Management, Swansea University, Wales, which provides educational programmes, research and consultancy in Value-Based Healthcare (VBHC), Value-Based Procurement (VBP) and Value-Based Supply (VBS). The Academy supports health systems and global life sciences companies to implement VBHC and to overcome the practical barriers to Value-Based Procurement by sharing learning and best practices around the World. The VBHC Academy is an expert affiliate to the EU Alliance for Value in Health, a member of the EFPIA VBHC Think-Tank, and works closely with MedTech Europe and the EU VBP Community of Practice.

Preface: Making Innovation Procurement Practical, Possible and Strategic

Carlos Larrañeta Gómez-Caminero

INTRODUCTION

At **Procure4Health**, we have always been strong believers in the potential of Innovation Procurement, especially in the health and care sector. From the beginning, it felt almost too good to be true: the idea that public procurement could go beyond administrative transactions to become a driver of system-wide transformation. What inspired us most was the persistent gap between innovation and implementation. New technologies continue to emerge, but without a reliable pathway into the healthcare system, much of their value is lost.

We also understood that healthcare is a complex ecosystem. Procurement does not occur in isolation: it requires coordination, communication and capability. So, our ambition was not only to demonstrate what Innovation Procurement can achieve but also to support those making it happen: the procurement professionals, project managers, clinicians, academics and policymakers working at the frontline of public healthcare systems. That is what Procure4Health set out to do: make Innovation Procurement not only possible but practical.

LEARNING BY DOING: OUR HANDS-ON APPROACH

From the outset, we embraced a highly practical approach. We knew this could not be a top-down exercise. Instead of simply developing guidelines or promoting policy frameworks, we focused on creating an environment where public buyers could test, adapt, and grow their capacity in real-world settings. The emphasis was always on learning by doing, grounded in real challenges and supported by peers across Europe.

Understanding who is in the room has been a cornerstone of our work. Not just institutions but individuals: what motivates them, where they encounter barriers and what kind of support makes a difference. This meant being flexible and adaptive, shaping processes to meet people where they are. It may sound simple, but this bottom-up responsiveness has been key to building trust and driving real change.

A STRATEGIC LEVER FOR SYSTEMIC CHANGE

Procure4Health has been a game-changer. Our aim was ambitious: to shift the mindset around public procurement from a transactional tool to a strategic lever for system-wide innovation. And we made it tangible. This wasn't just about producing reports; it was about building a living, breathing community of practice. A space where public buyers could learn from each other, develop shared tools and translate policy into action.

We connected more than 100 procuring entities from 24 countries, helping bridge the gap between local needs and European strategies. We created tools such as the Action Plan Template, the Early Demand Mapping methodology and the Twinning Programme, all designed to help regions move from one-off pilot projects to long-term, systemic strategies.

Our work addressed key health system priorities: sustainability, digital transformation, integrated care and personalised medicine. We placed a particular focus on practical implementation, enabling peer learning and fostering cross-functional collaboration.

INNOVATION AS A 3D PUZZLE: STRATEGY IN COMPLEX SYSTEMS

The ultimate goal of all our efforts has been clear: to ensure that new technological developments can be adopted effectively to improve the healthcare services provided to citizens. This is about continuous improvement, which inherently involves the ongoing adoption of innovation. And within the public sector, this means using the instrument of Public Procurement of Innovation (PPI) to make it happen.

Yet, we must be realistic. Public healthcare systems are complex structures, and driving innovation within them is like assembling a massive 3D puzzle. The individual pieces – strategy, operations, regulation and people – were never designed to fit together easily. And yet, they must.

Some of the critical components that must align include:

- *Defining and prioritising challenges*: We need to decide where to focus our efforts, knowing that resources are limited. This means evaluating potential value (short-, medium- and long-term), sustainability (environmental, financial, social) and strategic alignment (with existing policies, plans and programmes).
- *Ensuring corporate-level leadership*: Innovation cannot rely on individual enthusiasm alone. Key challenges should be defined by the end users; clinicians and patients, while prioritisation must be led by senior management, in collaboration with strategic and planning leads.
- *Enabling system-wide collaboration*: Successful innovation requires contributions from a wide range of actors who often do not naturally work together: patients, clinicians, technical staff (ICT, labs, infrastructure), legal and procurement teams, researchers, trainers and innovation officers.

On top of this, public buyers must navigate a demanding landscape of requirements, including:

- Compatibility with existing infrastructure.
- Compliance with GDPR, ethical standards and other regulatory frameworks.
- Public procurement legislation and European directives.
- Health technology assessments and evidence-based validation.
- The ability to engage fluently with solution providers.

Fitting all of these pieces together is no small task. Each healthcare system has its own size, structure, experience level and maturity. There is no one-size-fits-all model, but there is a shared need to equip people with the tools and confidence to act.

THE LEGACY: A STRONGER ECOSYSTEM AND A SHARED FOUNDATION

Looking ahead, the legacy of **Procure4Health** is twofold:

1. A strong and connected European network of innovation-driven public buyers.
2. A practical foundation of methods, tools and insights that others can now use to develop their own strategies.

The nine chapters that follow in this publication reflect that work. They offer hands-on guidance drawn from real experiences, covering the full lifecycle of Innovation Procurement: from challenge identification to value-based evaluation and sustainable implementation.

Our core recommendation? Invest in people. Innovation happens when we empower public buyers: not just with checklists and procedures, but with vision, capacity and trust. And above all: don't treat procurement as paperwork. Treat it as strategy.

1

Innovation Procurement – What is Innovation Procurement and Why is it Important?

Björn Lagnevik

INTRODUCTION

How do we create the solutions for tomorrow that are of great benefit for both humans and the environment? Innovation Procurement is a powerful, underused tool to drive change. Having worked within this field for 15 years, we share some of the most important points from these experiences.

Innovation Procurement has great potential to strengthen the renewal, quality and efficiency in public services in general and healthcare services, whilst at the same time having a positive impact on the innovativeness of industry towards sustainable growth. By using innovation and innovation-friendly procurement instruments for problem solving and not restricting public procurement to existing solutions, the unmet needs from procurers actively drive the development of new goods, services and processes.

If we restrict procurement methods to current or traditional practices, we will miss out on the innovative solutions provided by a competitive industry. Traditional methods of procurement tend to reward established larger suppliers and disadvantage small- and medium-enterprises (SMEs) and start-ups.

WHAT IS INNOVATION PROCUREMENT?

Public procurement is governed by and follows public laws and common tools and methodologies. Traditionally, public procurement focused on procuring existing products and services and the solutions being sought and requirements were therefore described in detail. If solutions can be described in the procurement documents, it is because they exist and, therefore, they cannot be regarded as innovations. If the products demanded by public agencies are described in technical terms, the procurer will get exactly those products – and not innovations. Hence, "regular procurement" is an obstacle to innovation. One cannot describe not-yet-existing products in advance.

Key in Innovation Procurement, as an alternative to regular procurement, is the emphasis the procuring organisation puts on describing the problems, missions or functions that the buyer wants to solve or fulfil, rather than listing technical specifications. When such a description exists, we use the term "functional procurement". Functional procurement is when a public agency buys products that perform functions that provide solutions to problems. In the case of functional procurement, the procuring organisation specifies *what* is to be achieved rather than *how*. Functional procurement can lead to new products (innovations) developed in the procurement process, and hence it creates opportunities for innovation. Moreover, not only does it cover the development of new state-of-the-art (SoTA) products but it can also be used in the deployment of innovative products with a high technology readiness level (TRL) but that are not yet available on the market through Public Procurement of Innovative Solutions (PPI). These innovations can, for example, contribute to saving the climate, saving the environment or curing diseases.

Innovation Procurement is when a public organisation publishes an unmet need or places an order for the fulfilment of certain functions by delivering, within a reasonable timescale, a new product (product, service or system) that does not exist at the time of the order, rather than product procurement. Innovation Procurement focuses on functions that satisfy human needs or solve health and/or social problems and not on stimulating the development of new products *per se*.

Procurement leading to innovations thus requires a functional description. If the functional description identifies that no solutions addressing the need are available on the market, the procurement leads to an innovation, or it may also lead to a

Figure 1.1 Innovation Procurement procedures

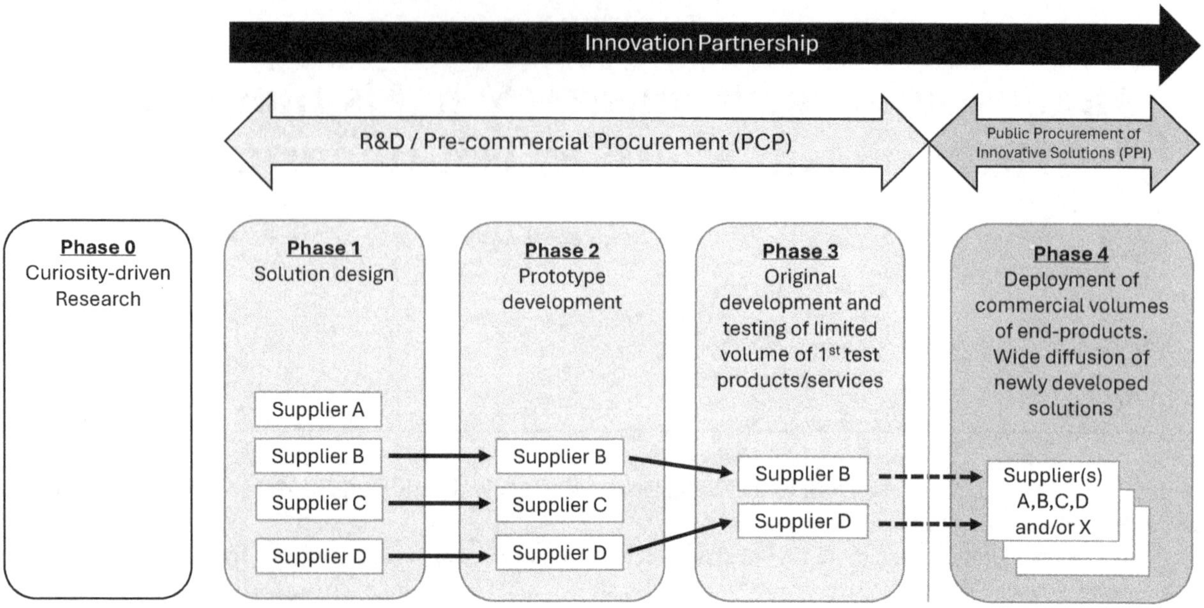

Source: Innovation Skåne

failure if no innovations result from the procurement process. However, if the functional description allows for the inclusion of products that already exist, then either the existing product or the new product can be procured.

Another example of this methodology is the so-called Innovation Partnership Procedure[1] to procure research and development (R&D) partners for a joint development project. Following the procurement of one or more suppliers, the companies develop new solutions in dialogue with the contracting organisation. If the results meet objectives regarding performance and costs, the solutions can be purchased directly from the procured companies/company, and a new procurement procedure is not needed. Companies can receive compensation for their development work in the project and, since the procurement is carried out in competition, the compensation may, if necessary, exceed what would have been possible in a state aid project.

This exemplifies that the term Innovation Procurement covers a range of procedures used by public procurers to solve societal challenges for which there are no existing solutions. In the European context, typical approaches are called Pre-Commercial Procurement (*PCP*) and *PPI.* According to DG CONNECT, PCP addresses the *development and testing* of innovative solutions, while PPI focuses on the *deployment* of innovative solutions.

COMMON FEATURES OF INNOVATION PROCUREMENT

Innovation Procurement typically will involve:

Competitive development in phases

Public procurers buy R&D from several competing suppliers in parallel to compare alternative solution approaches and identify the best value for money solutions that the market can deliver to address their needs. The R&D relationship is a collaborative one in which buyer and supplier can be described as co-developers of solutions addressing the unmet need. The procurement process is split into phases, with the number of competing R&D providers being reduced after each R&D phase.

1 While Procurement Innovation partnerships are regulated by procurement law, PCP and PPI are not.

Risk-benefit sharing under market conditions

Public procurers share the benefits and risks related to the Intellectual Property Rights (IPR) resulting from the R&D with suppliers at market price. Suppliers retain IPR ownership rights, while procurers keep some usage and licensing rights.

Separation from the deployment of commercial volumes of end-products/services

Specifically for the PCP procedure, and instrumental in the collaborative R&D relation between buyer and supplier, is the fact that the process goes up to the development and purchase of a limited volume of first products or services developed in the PCP ("limited" because, in a service contract like PCP, the total value of supplies purchased needs to remain below 50% of the total PCP contract value). As R&D cannot include quantity production (large-scale production to produce commercial volumes of end-products), PCP does not cover large-scale commercialisation. The deployment of commercial volumes of end-products is the remit of PPI. PCP is thus complementary to PPI.

Encouraging the creation of growth and jobs in Europe

Procedures fall outside of international public procurement agreements such as the World Trade Organisation (WTO) Agreement on Government Procurement [1]. Therefore, procedures can use "place of performance" conditions that require participating contractors to locate the majority of the activities performed for the contract, including in particular the principal staff working for the contract, in the EU Member States or associated countries. Examples of this can be seen in Horizon 2020 and Horizon Europe.

Different Levels of Innovation in Procurement

Different perspectives of innovation in procurement can be considered as a pyramid (figure 1.2). This indicates that there are three levels of Innovation Procurement with respect to their *innovativeness.*

Figure 1.2 Different perspectives and aspects of Innovation Procurement

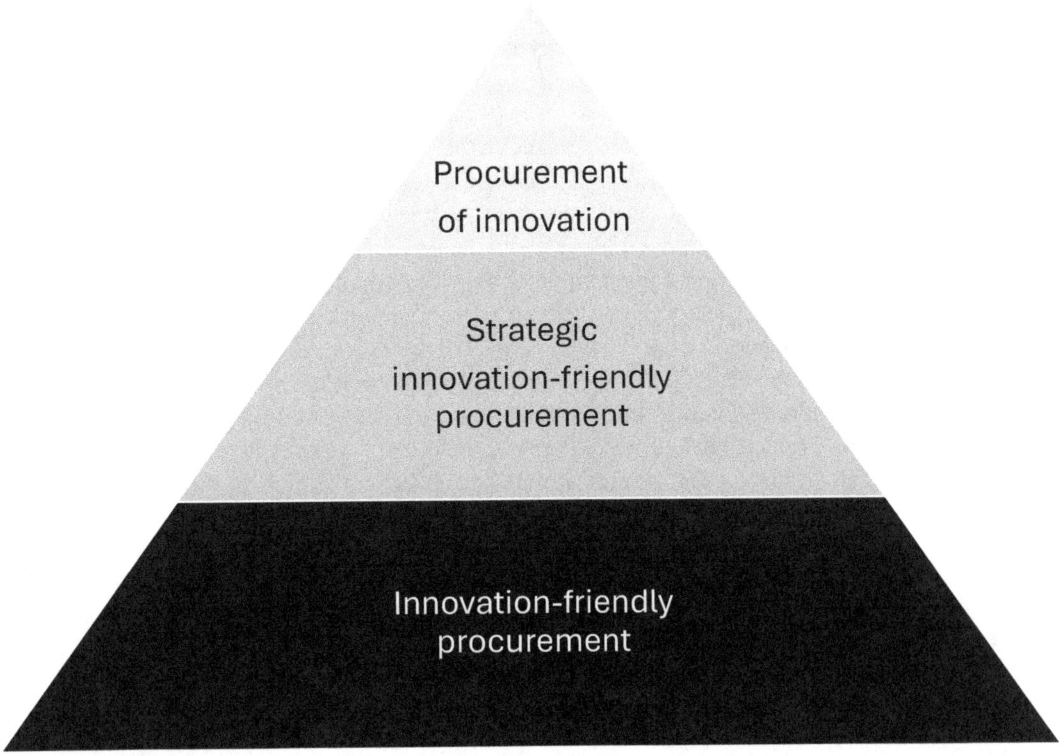

The top level, which has the greatest degree of innovativeness is **procurement of innovation**. When there are no solutions available, we can procure new solutions to solve our challenge or unmet need. The result is a new product or a new way of using an existing product.

The second level of the pyramid is **strategic innovation-friendly procurement**. This level is the middle segment regarding both the number of cases and degree of innovativeness. The result can be a new product within strategically important areas such as healthcare and environmental areas.

The base level is the largest part of the pyramid, which has the lowest level of innovativeness – **innovation-friendly procurement**. We define innovation-friendly procurement to be open towards new products and entrepreneurs. The result can be a new product purchased, but most likely it stimulates product development or alternative products.

THE IMPORTANCE OF INNOVATION PROCUREMENT

Innovation Procurement is potentially one of the more powerful innovation policy instruments currently available. It describes problems that shall be solved or functions that shall be fulfilled by means of procurement, rather than the products to be purchased. It works from the demand side, and it is powerful for two reasons. Firstly, the volume of public procurement is enormous (15% or more of global GDP), which is many times larger than the world expenditure on Research and Development! Secondly, this approach to public procurement can influence not only the speed, but also the direction of innovation processes.

If the products demanded by public agencies are described in technical terms, the procurer will get exactly those products – and not innovations. Hence, "regular procurement" is an obstacle to innovation. One cannot describe not-yet-existing products in advance. We have experienced great value in Innovation Procurement when we focused on functions and impact. The example of Region Skåne's work with bio-based medical aprons is given below.

When it comes to understanding the need for and development of Innovation Procurement, it is vital to create a process that enables innovation. There must be room for development during the innovation process, a sense of risk-sharing between involved partners and an openness to utilise different methods to unlock possibilities for different aims. Different aspects of Innovation Procurement that are highlighted include culture, organisation, strategy and adjustments of "regular procurement" to broaden the scope of innovation (and innovation-friendly) procurement. When including a broad range of different perspectives, allowing different methods to be used and adding strategic perspectives in addressing challenges, we are getting closer to Next Generation Procurement. When we have reached this far – we surely can address societal challenges through procurement methods.

Functional procurement is therefore particularly valuable in innovation policies whose objective it is to save the environment and climate – for example, by enhancing innovation processes in the direction of solar power instead of coal. Innovative procurement procedures have the potential to strengthen the renewal, quality and efficiency in public service provisioning, and at the same time, having a positive impact at the innovativeness of the industry towards sustainable growth. By using innovation and innovation-friendly procurement as instruments for problem solving and not restricting public procurement to existing solutions, public service demands actively can drive the development of new goods and services and new processes.

R&D collaboration refers to collaboration between public service providers and industry actors, with the goal of generating new knowledge and insights, and testing ideas. R&D collaboration does not directly lead to ready-made, marketable and implementable innovations in public services. There are clear advantages to engage in this type of R&D collaboration during exploration and early development. Close collaboration between healthcare and private actors ensures that, eventually, the appropriate solutions may be developed and offered on the market, based on the knowledge and insights generated from the project. Furthermore, it is relatively easy to start R&D collaboration projects, and a relatively large portion of public funding goes towards stimulating R&D collaboration. Co-development includes joint activities for the development and implementation of solutions not readily available on the market. The actors involved contribute with necessary unique skills and roles, and their responsibilities are clearly defined. Since co-development depends on the contribution of all involved actors, it may be possible to develop business models, agreements and contracts that reflect their respective contributions to the work. However, collaboration also presents complexity and difficult challenges for the actors involved; for example, to agree on common goals and expectations, as well as signing formal agreements.

As in the case of PCP, procurement can be used as a policy tool when a public procurer would like to stimulate R&D activities within a specific area. In using the PCP instrument in particular, the general rule is that project results generated are shared between procurer and supplier, the former primarily acquiring knowledge for preparations of future procured products, rather than a final solution. It is important to be able to prove that collaboration really concerns R&D and, if this is the case, that R&D collaboration is exempt from procurement legislation. However, sometimes it is still advisable to carry out a procurement to select and secure the most competent R&D partner, and to ensure an open and transparent process.

To ensure that co-development is the right approach to choose, a thorough analysis of the wider context, that is, business intelligence and market analysis, is required, and a broad market dialogue is recommended. It is important to understand if solutions are available or not in the market, but also that the market is sufficiently mature, so that development of a final solution is possible.

The Swedish agency for innovation Vinnova's report "Innovation Power in the Public Sector" [2] states that innovation within, and in collaboration with public authorities, plays an important role for the development and growth of society. Public sector revenue in Sweden alone accounts for almost 50% of the Swedish GDP and procurements amount to more than SEK 700 billion/year.

The report further highlights several barriers for innovation within the public sector: time and money but also a "lack of knowledge on how to actually do it". Leadership is considered critical to successful innovation work, as is the need for support for a more structured and systematic way of working with innovation from idea to implementation and adoption. The report also emphasises the importance of avoiding the "project trap"; that is, developing solutions that only facilitate specific project deliverables, but which are not possible to implement and introduce into regular practice after the project is completed.

Public/Private Collaboration and a Healthy Innovation Ecosystem

The OECD (Organisation for Economic Cooperation and Development) states that public healthcare providers can do more to use their innovation strengths to stimulate growth and employment generation and that greater private sector involvement in the innovation system is needed. Furthermore, OECD states these providers can move from research and technology hubs towards wealthy and inclusive innovative regions. OECD identifies common shortcomings in regional health and care ecosystems to be lack of entrepreneurs and entrepreneurship; new firms remain small and there is a dependence on a few larger companies (if any).

A Strategic Instrument for Growth, Resilience and Cutting-Edge Research

The process of capturing an innovation and being able to deploy it through a series of strictly defined process steps can be illustrated as below, and this relates closely to procurement (and adoption) of innovations.

Public investment and innovation are two essential ways to meet the challenges of the recovery, the green and digital transition and the creation of a more resilient economy in the EU. The new Recovery and Resilience Facility will drive public investment after the COVID crisis, and a large part of this investment will be channelled through public procurement. EU benchmarking shows that Europe is exploiting only half of the potential power of Innovation Procurement to fuel economic recovery and that there is large underinvestment, particularly in the procurement of digital solutions and in R&D procurement, both of which are key for strengthening the EU's strategic autonomy and competitiveness. Public buyers will need to boost Innovation Procurement and help businesses to develop innovative solutions in key industrial ecosystems, in especially where public buyers are critical investors. Public buyers will also have to foster the resilience of the European economy by diversifying sources of supply in essential commodities, such as pharmaceutical ingredients, as revealed by the COVID-19 pandemic, and by promoting new solutions.

The use of Innovation Procurement by public authorities at national, regional and local levels can greatly contribute to the implementation of the green deal and the digitalisation of the interaction between companies/citizens and public administrations. It also creates considerable potential for cross-border cooperation.

Figure 1.3 Capturing innovation through the innovation cycle [3]

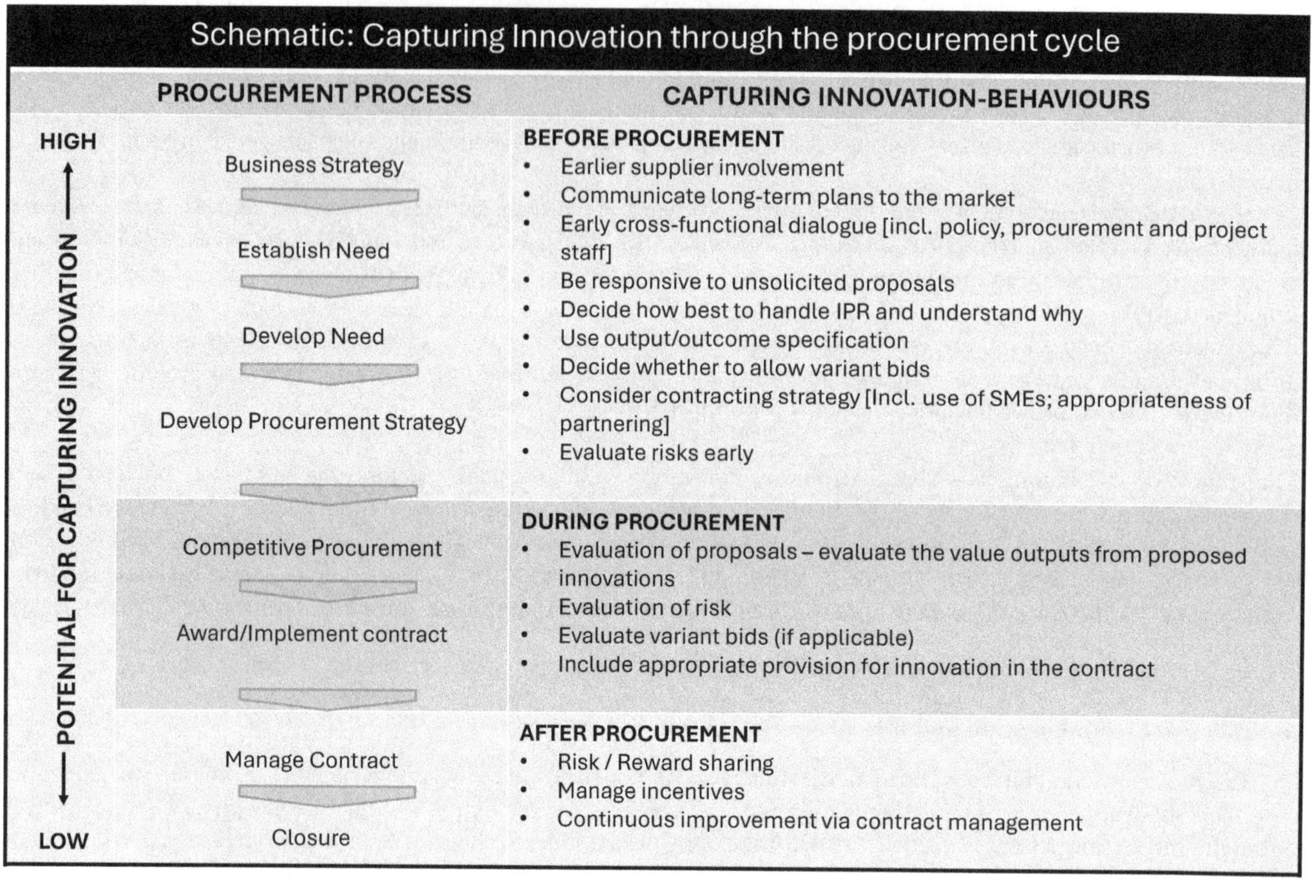

GUIDING PRINCIPLES

Unmet Needs in the Front Seat

Public procurement accounts for a very large share of most economies worldwide, and key to achieving more innovations is the process of describing the problems to be solved or functions to be fulfilled instead of describing the products to be bought (regular procurement). Contracting authorities need to identify the problems that policy should address. Innovations solving the problems are then designed by the potential innovators/suppliers, not by public procurers. Therefore, the societal needs and problems must be translated and transformed into functional requirements. Functional procurement is allowed in European regulations and so there are no legal obstacles to using it for innovation policy purposes. Furthermore, it leads to increased competition, not only among potential suppliers of similar products, but also among different products that solve the same problem.

Before drafting technical specifications, public buyers should perform a wide-ranging needs assessment to define the problem that is to be solved. This step may seem superfluous, as the purpose of the public procurement procedure is usually obvious. In fact, this is the crucial moment when innovation uptake may originate. Instead of simply replacing outdated equipment with more of the same, or renewing expired service contracts, the public buyer carries out a functional analysis of the needs of the organisation and its partners/users and identifies any problems or areas for improvement. This analysis will reveal whether the equipment and services used until now are (still) the most appropriate ones.

The definition of needs requires keeping an adequate distance from the current solution to assess it with maximum impartiality. It is important to keep an open mind about introducing modifications or replacing the existing solutions altogether. In some cases, a deep organisational change may be required, especially if workflows have been automated. In practice, the needs assessment may lead to considering a different type of contract than the existing one with the incumbent; that is, instead of supply contract, a service contract or a mixed (supply and service) contract may be more appropriate for the new technologies or processes. To allow new trends or exploit technological advantages that public buyers are not aware of yet, market(s) shall be screened. Public buyers might discover new, innovative solutions to provide public services, to increase service levels or add additional functions by using new technologies. Thus, public buyers can tailor their needs based on a thorough understanding of the market, which also enables them to incorporate innovative solutions into the procurement process.

A Creative Mindset and Collaborative Culture

To succeed in Innovation Procurement and innovation-friendly procurement, a changed mindset is crucial. Curiosity is key – towards, for instance, entrepreneurs and their conditions. Courage is required to try new methods and to decrease the detailed requirements on our suppliers and the goods and services we procure. It is fairly obvious that regular procurement is easier and lower risk than Innovation Procurement. This applies for both contracting authorities and employees. Risk aversion within decision makers and contracting authorities reduces the tendency to follow Innovation Procurement processes.

Openness and dialogue

By using dialogue, we acquire knowledge about the market, the suppliers operating in it and the kind of solutions they offer. We also learn about current state-of-the-art and new trends. Moreover, we can learn about other relevant markets and value chains to find technologies and processes which may be transferred.

Through dialogue, we get input from entrepreneurs about our needs and the way we could procure, and we also stimulate enterprises to tender for our specific procurements, resulting in increased competition. Since the tenderers understand the public service providers' unmet needs better, the tenders are also improved and more relevant. Inviting potential suppliers into early dialogue is also a way of increasing transparency and improving long-term relations with industry actors.

Figure 1.4 Dialogue Process Cycle

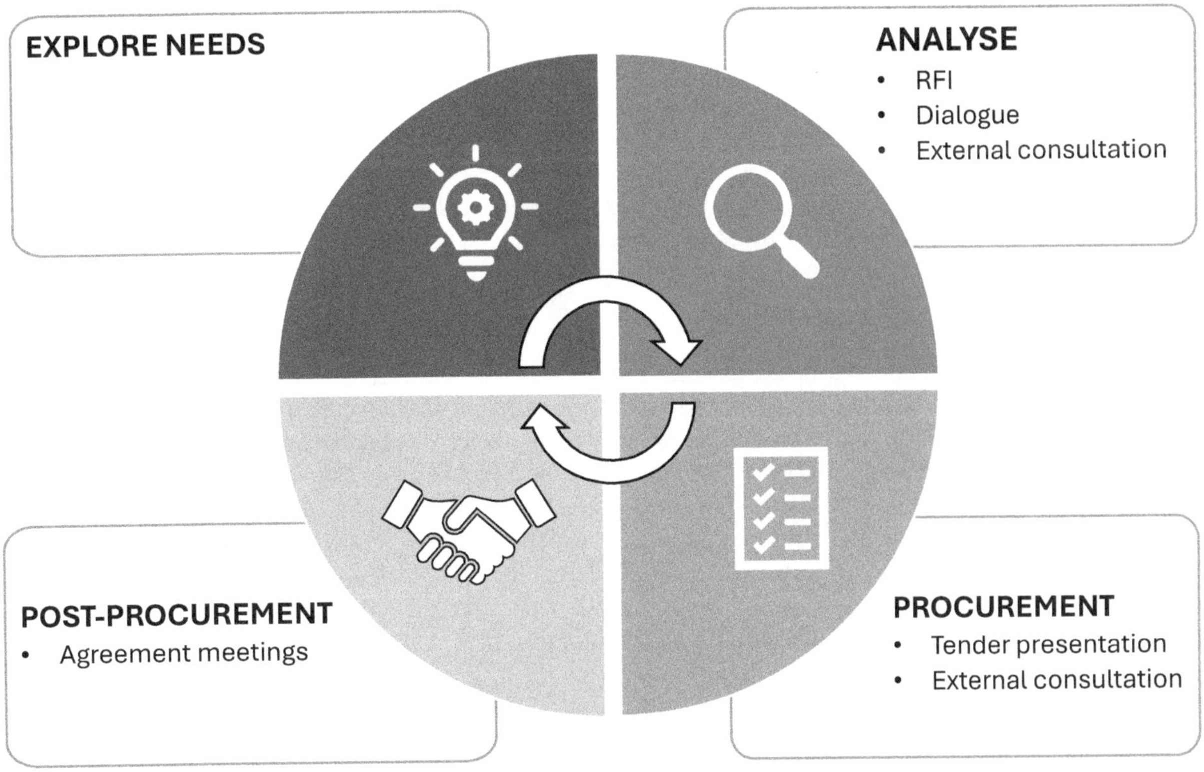

DIALOGUE PROCESS

Dialogue or interaction with different kinds of actors in the market is essential to be innovation-friendly – without any interaction, there will be no innovation. This is an important element of effective procurement strategies. Any dialogue or interaction that fulfils the principles for public procurement in the legislation should be considered. This is important throughout the different phases of the procurement process. Dialogue should be used before, during and after the specific procurements, but it can also be used without connection to a specific procurement; therefore, there are several opportunities to use this tool. However, even if the impact of dialogue is very high, there are not infinite resources available and so we should try to use dialogue smartly. The more important the strategic objective is, the more dialogue we should undertake, and we should also choose the most effective form for each scenario.

Before Initiating the Procurement Process

By using dialogue, we get good knowledge about the market, with information about enterprises in that market and what kind of solutions they offer. We also look for information about new trends and what solutions are under development. We should also try to investigate other markets to find solutions that have the potential to be transferable.

Dialogue will stimulate lots of inputs from entrepreneurs in response to our needs and the ways we could procure. Some of these inputs are of great value but some of them are, of course, more marketing by the enterprise, and this should be kept in mind. By using dialogue, we also stimulate enterprises to submit late tenders for specific procurements. In this way, dialogue increases competition, leading to better deals for the procuring party in the end. Since the tenderers gain a better understanding of our needs, the later tenders are usually of a higher quality. Inviting potential suppliers into dialogue also increases transparency and improves long-term relations with enterprises.

Dialogue During the Procurement

This procurement phase is characterised by a low level of external interaction. There is some potential for increasing interaction – for instance, for the purposes of promoting the tender, through outreach to supplier networks, etc. The main restriction is the risk of acting against the principles of equal treatment of the tenderers, which must be respected.

Dialogue After the Procurement

After the award decision has been made, the tenderers can be invited for a vendor debriefing meeting. The purpose of the meeting is to get feedback about how to improve the process. It is an opportunity for the procuring organisation to improve its processes and be more innovation-friendly. It is also an opportunity to present some feedback about the individual tender.

It is also important to have a continuous active dialogue between the buyer and the supplier during the agreement period. The focus in this phase is to follow up and to develop the contract.

CLOSING REMARKS

Our take-home message when it comes to understanding the need for, and development of, Innovation Procurement is to create a process that enables innovation to take place. There must be room for development during the innovation process, a sense of risk sharing between involved partners and openness for different methods to unlock possibilities for different aims. The different aspects of Innovation Procurement that are highlighted include: culture, organisation, strategy and adjustments of "regular procurement" to broaden the scope of innovation (and innovation-friendly) procurement. When including a broad range of different perspectives, allowing different methods to be used and adding strategic perspectives in addressing challenges, we are getting closer to Next Generation Procurement. When we have reached this point, we can then say that we can address societal challenges through procurement methods.

EXAMPLE OF INNOVATION PROCUREMENT IN HEALTH

Disposable bio-based aprons for Skåne's healthcare sector (Sweden)

Following an analysis carried out in 2011 of the Region of Skåne's impacts on climate change emissions, the regional council discovered that 40% of the Skåne's CO_2 emissions were generated through its healthcare sector. A large part of this impact was caused by single-use (or disposable) products, such as protective aprons. In 2014, Skåne's healthcare sector was responsible for using and disposing of 5.2 million single-use aprons, generating the equivalent of 300 tonnes of CO_2 emissions. The climate impact caused by these kinds of products can be reduced by limiting unnecessary consumption, finding new materials offering better performance and lower weight, as well as replacing fossil-based materials with fossil-free alternatives through, for example, Innovation Procurement.

As a climate-neutral disposable protective apron was not available on the market at that time, the Region of Skåne embarked on an innovation-oriented public procurement process to purchase aprons mostly made from renewable (bio-based) material. The process began in 2014 and concluded in May 2016, with the contract awarded to a company for the supply of disposable aprons consisting of 91% renewable material. The purchase/use of the bio-based aprons is expected to result in savings of 250 tonnes per year of CO_2 emissions.

For the Region of Skåne, the procurement exercise meant not only that it was possible to stimulate innovation, which led to the development of a more climate-neutral product, but that it was also possible to create a model for how a PPI can be implemented, with lessons – and newly developed materials – that can be implemented in future procurement processes. The spin-off effects of the procurement are worthy of note; it facilitated a large demand from other public bodies, created fifteen jobs and dissemination to related areas with many disposable products.

REFERENCES

1. World Trade Organisation (WTO) Agreement on Government Procurement. https://www.wto.org/english/tratop_e/gproc_e/gp_gpa_e.htm
2. Vinnova: The innovative power of public enterprise (2020). https://www.vinnova.se/en/publikationer/the-innovative-power-of-public-enterprise/
3. EC-RTD, Developing procurement practices favourable to R&D and innovation (2005). https://ec.europa.eu/invest-in-research/pdf/download_en/edited_report_18112005_on_public_procurement_for_research_and_innovation.pdf

FURTHER READING

EC Guidance on Innovation Procurement (2021). https://eur-lex.europa.eu/legal-content/EN/TXT/PDF/?uri=CELEX:52021XC0706(03)&from=EN

Functional procurement for innovation, welfare, and the environment (Edquist, Zabala-Iturriagagoitia) (2020). https://charlesedquist.files.wordpress.com/2021/04/edquist_zabala-iturriagagoitia_scipol2020.pdf

Borgegård T, Persson S, Mårtensson Djäken E, Gustafsson T. The game plan for development and innovation within public healthcare (2021). https://swelife.se/wp-content/uploads/2021/01/Game-Plan-Sweper-brochure-ENG-20201015.pdf

Public Sector Innovation – the case of Sweden (2020). https://www.vinnova.se/contentassets/9fab4046146e48379590a157481d3d7d/vr20-02eng.pdf

2

The Process of Innovation Procurement

Key Steps and Existing Instruments

Diana Cortés Rodríguez

INTRODUCTION

Public procurement enables provision of basic services, such as healthcare, infrastructure and energy. Healthcare is the second largest spending area for governments, representing over 9% of GDP [1]. Public Procurement of Innovation (PPI) is a key instrument not only for public investment but also for economic development in general. Public procurement/demand-driven innovation can open markets for industry/researchers creating growth and jobs in Europe. It is a methodology that introduces new opportunities into the market, fostering for the first time the demand for innovative products that are incipient in research centres, and creating new business opportunities between start-ups and companies already established in the productive sector. This is why Innovation Procurement is considered a public policy strategy that favours the creation of synergies within the market and stimulates investment by private sector agents in the public administration, thus establishing a new path for job creation.

Although Public Procurement of Innovation is a very powerful instrument for fostering innovation, it is important to bear in mind that, depending on the strategic priorities of the region or country, different types of public procurement can be defined and configured (Pre-Commercial Public Procurement, Public Procurement of Innovative Solutions and Innovation Partnership). Based on our experience, any Public Procurement of Innovation project should follow a series of stages to be developed successfully, including the shaping of the project idea, validation of the unmet needs, Open Market Consultation (OMC), funding opportunities identification, the launch of the Public Procurement of Innovation tender, the award of the contract(s), its implementation and closure. These stages are the main points that will be described.

Public Procurement of Innovative solutions happens when the public sector uses its purchasing power to act as an early adopter of innovative solutions that are not yet available on a large-scale commercial basis. Public procurement refers to the purchase by governments and state-owned enterprises of goods, services and works in a sequence of activities, starting with the assessment of needs through awards to contract management and final payment.

This chapter focuses primarily on the current Public Procurement of Innovation framework, its context (legal, policy, social, etc.) and available instruments. One of the key parts is a description of the Public Procurement of Innovation roadmap, including the preparatory tasks (identification of unmet needs, Open Market Consultation), the project design and allocation of the different Public Procurement of Innovation instruments; the identification of funding opportunities, the tender development, contracts awarding, project monitoring and management. Thus, the key stages of the process are highlighted, including information about the different steps to be developed, from the project award to the necessary organisational change management to adopt Innovation Procurement.

Coordination between all the actors involved in an Innovation Procurement project is essential to ensure the success of these projects. Therefore, Public Procurement of Innovation is configured as an appropriate instrument for "ecosystem creation" of knowledge around the public demand for products and services. Given the ambition and impact of Public Procurement of Innovation projects, there is usually a wide range of stakeholders involved in the design and development of PPI projects.

PUBLIC PROCUREMENT OF INNOVATION: KEY CONCEPTS AND OBJECTIVES

According to the Directive 2014/24/EU, Public Procurement of Innovation is the implementation of a new or significantly improved product, service or process, including but not limited to production, building or construction processes, a new marketing method or a new organisational method in business practices, workplace organisation or external relations *inter alia*, with the purpose of helping to solve societal challenges or to support the Europe 2020 strategy for smart, sustainable and inclusive growth.

Public procurement refers to the purchase by governments and state-owned enterprises of goods, services and works. As public procurement accounts for a substantial proportion of taxpayers' money, governments are expected to carry it out efficiently and with high standards of conduct to ensure high quality of service delivery and safeguard the public interest.

The public sector is faced with important challenges. Addressing these often requires public sector transformation. In many cases, solutions are close to market and would be provided if clear requirements and/or sufficient demand were expressed by the market. In other cases, R&D is still required to de-risk technology and competing solutions need to be compared before committing to large-scale deployment.

To achieve this several instruments have been designed and used. Following are three such instruments.

Pre-Commercial Public Procurement [3]

PCP consists of procuring research and development services with advantageous conditions from several economic operators. Its objective is to steer the development of solutions towards clearly defined public sector needs, whilst comparing/validating alternative solution approaches from various vendors. It can be used when there are not yet near-to-the-market solutions and new R&D is needed. PCP can then compare the pros and cons of alternative competing solution approaches. This will in turn de-risk the most promising innovations step-by-step via solution design, prototyping, development and first product testing.

Public Procurement of Innovative Solutions

PPIs objective is to act to launch customer/early adopter/first buyer of innovative commercial end-solutions newly arriving on the market. It is used when challenges can be addressed by innovative solutions that are nearly or already in the market in small quantities and do not need new R&D.

Innovation Partnership [4]

The aim of an innovation partnership is to develop "an innovative product, service or work and to subsequently purchase" the resulting supplies, services or works' providing that they correspond to the performance levels and maximum costs agreed between the contracting authority and the participants.

EU's research and innovation programmes have been funding projects in which groups of procurers from different countries around Europe are jointly implementing PCP or PPIs, as well as coordination and networking projects that prepare the ground for future PCP or PPIs. As an example, there is a list of projects in the ICT domain, most of them in the Digital Health field [5].

CONTEXT OF PUBLIC PROCUREMENT OF INNOVATION: LEGAL, POLICY, SOCIAL, FINANCIAL, TECHNICAL AND COMPETENCE

It is important to identify the potential limits that can be found for the adoption of Public Procurement of Innovation in the health and social care sector. For that, several challenges and barriers have been summarised and classified in the following areas.

Legal and Policy

Public Procurement of Innovation may differ from more conventional public procurements and require thorough procurement control and audit processes. This can make the process burdensome due to bureaucracy inertia and a lack of knowledge regarding PPI. A key point also is to guarantee real commitment to extend the project beyond the pilot stage from all the different actors in the project. Concerning Digital Health, it implies more market uncertainty as there is a need for further evaluation regarding the innovation solutions compared with other sectors and there is also a regulatory gap [6]. Related to this, innovation usually goes hand-in-hand with uncertainty and risk. Therefore, there is a need to create a formal and standardised system to ensure that public procurement of innovative products and services is transparent and accountable. This system should include clear guidelines and procedures for the selection, evaluation and award of contracts.

Social

The political environment does not fully support Public Procurement of Innovation as, often, there are no clear targets in all EU countries, and a lack of understanding of the instrument, the bureaucracy, uncertainty and risk of innovation projects. For Health and Social Care, human-centric product development should be considered to ensure that the health and social care technology tools that are being brought to market address the unmet needs of the users. Procurers need to promote public awareness and education of the Public Procurement of Innovation process and the benefits of investing in innovative products and services and should give feedback and evaluation to stakeholders to ensure that the public procurement process is effective and efficient.

Financial

R&D projects rarely focus on commercialisation, which risks subsequent commercial failure. The geopolitical context is complex and uncertain, although the EC has activated a massive package of funds to combat various crises (COVID-19, the war in Ukraine, energy-price drawbacks), it is unclear how this will affect investment in R&D and innovation and thus the administration has taken a step back in the planning and allocation of resources to Public Procurement of Innovation projects. For Health and Social Care there is a need to fund continued investment in hands-on training to improve technology literacy of patients, social care and healthcare professionals and providers. When focusing on Digital Health, there is still limited large-scale evidence of the cost-effectiveness of these tools and services.

Technical and Competence

There are several issues to be addressed. Interoperability between different equipment and between different social care and health systems and services providers continues to be a major challenge. The use of Big Data is constrained because health information is highly sensitive. The privacy and protection of user data is a security concern. The fast-changing nature of technology can be problematic and there is a lack of transparency regarding the utilisation of data collected by Digital Health applications. A common demand within the social care and health community is the need to develop validated solutions. Data protection should be included as a standard in all procurement processes. Innovation Procurement is one way of understanding (from the buyer's side) all technical aspects from a clearer perspective and in a more responsive, accurate and up-to-date way by providing descriptions of the technical perspective and current State-of-the-Art (SoTA).

At the same time, some challenges associated with the implementation of Public Procurement must be considered. Unmet needs, and the failure to identify them until they become urgent problems, are incompatible with Procurement of Innovation practices. Urgent-base-working schemes should also be avoided, and unmet needs identification cannot be tackled in non-collaborative environments. During the implementation of the process, the fear of change, user resistance and risk aversion are key factors to assess.

When talking about opportunities related to unmet needs, we refer to encouraging the market by developing early demand maps, promote institutional and possibly financial support for "matchmaking". This match should be between scientific institutions and companies, creating capacity for the identification of unmet needs oriented to Public Procurement of Innovation projects, with staff trained and motivated to emphasise Public Procurement of Innovation joint actions and collaboration schemes.

In opportunities related to the implementation process, different key agents such as Social Care and Health organisations within the EU Member States could contribute by providing additional tools, data, and methodologies/guidelines for specific policy or geographical areas, thus creating a community of users that will maximise its reuse. Also, supportive guidelines, standards and accreditation schemes could be developed for the Digital Health technologies, tools and services under development.

For procurers, it is essential that they improve their technical skills, have know-how in supply chain management and gain a better understanding of Public Procurement of Innovation mechanisms. Suppliers need to increase their competences in Public Procurement of Innovation and emphasise implementation and promoting the creation of Innovation ecosystems to foster local innovation and growth.

PUBLIC PROCUREMENT OF INNOVATION ROADMAP

Preparatory Tasks: Unmet Needs and Open Market Consultation

This first stage comprises the high-level design of the project, starting from the assessment of the challenge or need to be covered. During the phases prior to the launch of a tender, it is considered that the key is to establish a fluid dialogue between the different areas of the competent administration; the owners of the needs and future project managers and the members of the coordination office (whose aim is the coordination of all the actors involved), to seek effective coordination for the definition of the needs and the functional requirements of the future project.

If the agents promoting the need do not have the necessary experience and/or resources of its own, the coordination office will be responsible for advising on the process of management and analysis of the needs for the configuration of the PPI challenge. Usually, the starting point for the configuration of a PPI project is an agent who identifies a need to improve the public service it provides. To outline this need, it is a common practice to work with standard forms that will help to assess its relevance and priority, the state of the art of the technology and the resources potentially available to carry it out (human resources, budget, etc.). This implies involvement of a broader perspective and actors for a more comprehensive overview of the challenge.

The next step will be the validation of the need with the group of agents that are part of the ecosystem of action around the need. Among the validation strategies and activities, the organisation of events aimed at contrasting the needs with the different profiles involved, also known as "focus groups", stands out. These events may involve, for example, associations, patients, groups of expert professionals, etc., depending on the field of action in each case. During these actions, dynamics should be applied that are specifically aimed at raising ideas and prioritising them (creativity sessions, ideation, consensus, etc.) to help shape the challenges.

Organising this type of pooling meetings with members of the ecosystem (citizens, representatives of the academic sector, etc.) will significantly enrich the validation and specification of needs, the analysis of solutions in use, and the development of the challenge(s). The information gathered in the events or focus groups should be used to prioritise/deprioritise, validate or reorient the information initially provided in the PPI project fiche.

Open Market Consultation

The OMC process comprises the analysis of the availability, scope, newness, technical and economic feasibility and functional performance of possible alternative solutions that respond to the needs and challenges posed, to address the unmet needs as current available products are insufficient. The next step will be to draw up a report on the conclusions and closure of the OMC, which the contracting body will make public. This report shall contain at least the following information:

1. Description of the challenge.
2. OMC Procedure.
3. Results of the OMC.
4. Technical conclusions.
5. Administrative conclusions.
6. Early Demand Map: The Early Demand Map is a document that contains a list of those needs in which the Public Procurement of Innovation modality would provide a way to satisfy them, because their procurement through conventional contracting procedures would not fit. As this is an instrument that allows the market to be informed of the needs of the Administration, it provides valuable information to companies to guide their R&D and Innovation initiatives towards possible tenders.

Project Design: PCP, PPIs and Innovation Partnership

This stage comprises the design and implementation of a Public Procurement of Innovation project, taking the results of the OMC as a starting point.

First it is important to analyse the legal and technical characteristics of the different procurement procedures based on a rigorous analysis of all the information resulting from the OMC, and considering the following key aspects:

- Establishment of the baseline and the target scenario regarding the identified challenge.
- Assessment of this baseline and target TRLs based on the results of the OMC.

Table 2.1 Technology Readiness Level (TRL)

TRL 9:	Actual system "flight proven" through successful mission operations
TRL 8:	Actual system completed and "flight qualified" through test and demonstration
TRL 7:	System prototype demonstration in a space environment
TRL 6:	System/subsystem model or prototype demonstration in a relevant environment
TRL 5:	Component and/or breedboard validation in relevant environment
TRL 4:	Component and/or breedboard validation in laboratory environment
TRL 3:	Analytical and experimental critical function and/or characteristic proof-of-concept
TRL 2:	Technology concept and/or application formulated
TRL 1:	Basic principles observed and reported

Source: NASA

Table 2.2 Summary of advantages and disadvantages of the different Public Procurement of Innovation procedures

Type	**TRL**	**Advantages**	**Disadvantages**
PCP	TRL 1–7	• Procedural flexibility • Favours the management of IPRs • Good control of R&D uncertainty	• Generates legal uncertainty • Necessarily pre-commercial results
PPIs	TRL 6–8	• Legal certainty • Commercial products • Standard procedures	• Restrictions in terms of award procedures
Innovation Partnership	TRL 1–8	• A single act to award R&D and supply • Good control of R&D uncertainty	• Complexity in developing the specifications • (especially in terms of performance for transition to supply)

Source: SILO Company

- Assessment of the need to request additional technology watch documents to deepen the analysis of the state of the art of the technology.
- Assessment of the need to consult internal or external experts on the technology.
- Assessment of the need to consult the companies again to clarify any point or issue that is considered key (by reopening the consultations if they had been closed).
- Evaluation of the cost-benefit ratio of each project and the economic impact of having a new innovative solution in terms of efficiency, effectiveness, and availability.
- For all procurement phases, it is desirable in the design process to enable time for reflection and dialogue.

The definition of the Public Procurement of Innovation typology (table 2.1) is based on the TRL scale, developed by NASA [7] for the standardisation of the assessment of the closeness to market of a technology, and adopted as a standard by the European Commission.

Technology Readiness Levels are a type of measurement system used to assess the maturity level of a particular technology. Each technology project is evaluated against the parameters for each technology level and is then assigned a TRL rating based on the project's progress. There are nine technology readiness levels. TRL 1 is the lowest and TRL 9 is the highest.

Once the TRL has been established, advice can be given on the most suitable PPI alternative, assessing the pros and cons of each option, followed by a detailed analysis.

In Table 2.2, the different procurement procedures are identified with the advantages and disadvantages of each of them and the TRL level range:

IDENTIFICATION OF FUNDING OPPORTUNITIES

Contracting Authority's Own Funds

These are the sources that come mainly from the budgets of the corresponding Public Administration, as well as from the different options available (extending the useful life of assets, financing future savings, etc.).

Next-Generation EU [8]

A temporary recovery instrument that will help repair the immediate economic and social damage caused by the coronavirus pandemic:

- *Recovery and Resilience Facility:* This is a central element of Next Generation EU, with loans and grants available to support reforms and investments undertaken by EU countries. The aim is to mitigate the economic and social impact of the coronavirus pandemic and to make European economies and societies more sustainable and resilient and better prepared for the challenges and opportunities of the green and digital transitions.
- *Recovery Assistance for Europe's Cohesion and Territories (REACT-EU):* This is a new initiative that continues and extends the crisis response and repair measures implemented through the Coronavirus Response Investment Initiative and the Coronavirus Response Investment Initiative Plus. It will contribute to a green, digital and resilient recovery of the economy.

ERDF: European Regional Development Fund [9]

Cohesion policy addresses a variety of development needs in all EU regions and cities. The European Structural and Investment Funds (ESIF) include several types of funds (ERDF, CF, ESF+, EAFRD, EMFF, FJT, etc.). The European Regional Development Fund (ERDF) provides funding to public and private bodies in all EU regions to reduce economic, social and territorial disparities. The ERDF supports investments through specific national or regional programmes.

In 2021–2027, the Fund will enable investment to make Europe and its regions:

- Become more competitive and smarter, through innovation and support for SMEs, as well as digitisation and digital connectivity.
- Greener, low-carbon and resilient.
- More connected by improving mobility.
- More social, supporting effective and inclusive employment, education, skills, social inclusion and equal access to healthcare, as well as enhancing the role of culture and sustainable tourism.
- Be closer to citizens, supporting local development and sustainable urban development across the EU.

Horizon Europe and Other

Horizon Europe [10] is the EU's ambitious Framework Programme for Research and Innovation (2021–2027) to strengthen the EU's scientific and technological foundations and the European Research Area (ERA), to boost Europe's innovation capacity, competitiveness and jobs and to deliver on citizens' priorities and to sustain our values and socio-economic model.

Horizon Europe has a budget of €95.5bn, making it the largest transnational research and innovation programme in the world. The programme is organised around three pillars and six clusters, which aim to cover the strategic points of action defined by the Commission.

HaDEA [11]

HaDEA manages calls for proposals and calls for tenders, which are open to a variety of organisations, including health NGOs and national authorities from EU countries and non-EU countries associated with the programme. HaDEA implements most of EU4Health, the largest programme to boost health around the EU, by managing calls for proposals and tenders from 2021 to 2027.

Figure 2.1 Horizon Europe, structure and budget.

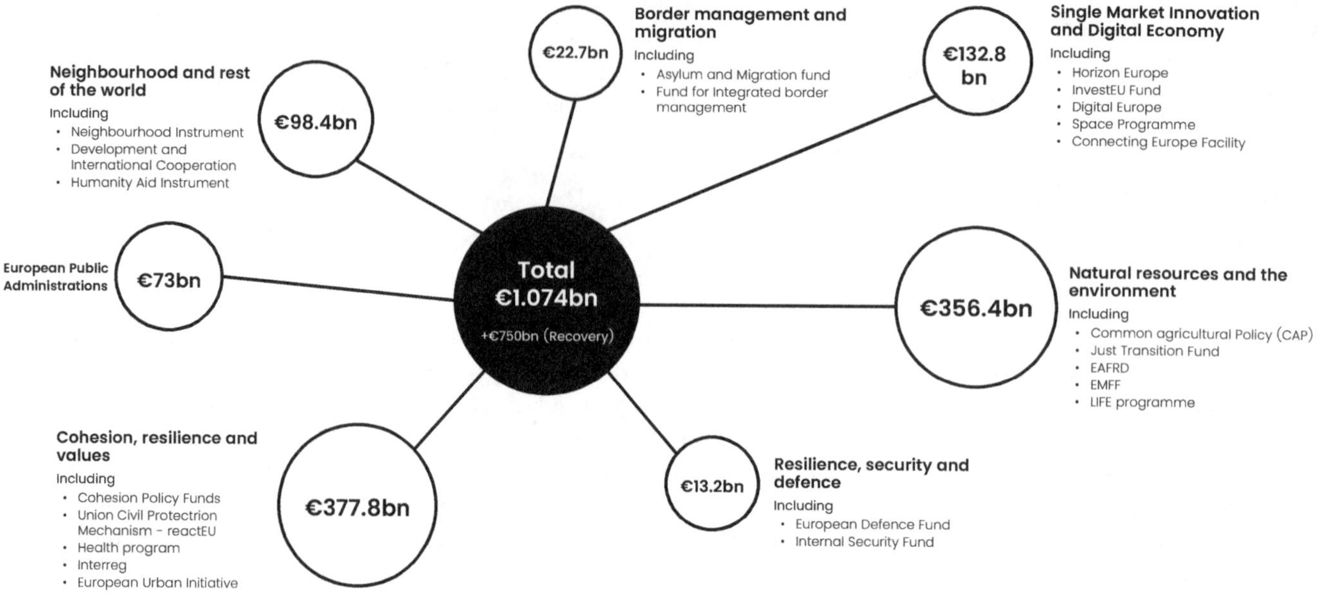

Source: SILO Company

EU4Health [12]

EU4Health is the EU's largest health programme in monetary terms, with a budget of €5.3 billion in current prices. The EU4Health programme goes beyond an ambitious response to the COVID-19 crisis to address the resilience of European healthcare systems. EU4Health provides funding to national authorities, health organisations and other bodies through grants and public procurement, contributing to a healthier Europe. The EU4Health programme also funds joint actions managed by competent national authorities. It is implemented through annual work programmes, which for 2023 consisted of four overarching strands: crisis preparedness, health promotion and disease prevention, health systems and healthcare workforce and digital. Also, Cancer is considered a fifth cross-cutting strand.

Interreg Europe [13]

Interreg promotes transnational cooperation to address issues common to the regions of the territory, such as low investment in research and development, low competitiveness of small- and medium-sized enterprises and exposure to climate change and environmental risks.

For the period 2021–2027, this programme has been endowed with nearly 10,000 million euros, marking the next step of Interreg towards a reinforced model of cooperation between EU member countries and their allies through Interreg IPA, Interreg NEXT and the integration of a line specifically dedicated to cooperation with the countries of the most remote regions of Europe.

Interreg is organised into separate strands:

- Interreg strand A: Cross Border Cooperation: It seeks to promote collaboration between European countries and with their closest neighbours.
- Interreg Strand B: Transnational Cooperation: This includes programmes aimed at collaboration between specific regions that share geographical areas.
- Interreg Strand C: Interregional Cooperation: Promotes the improvement in the efficiency of cohesion policy through the exchange of experiences, innovative approaches and capacity building between regions.

DEVELOPMENT OF THE PROCUREMENT OF INNOVATION TENDER

The objective of this phase is the drafting and processing of the documents and specifications, as well as the launching of the Public Procurement of Innovation tender. It includes everything from the beginning of the procurement file to its approval by the contracting entity. It usually involves the following units and profiles: promoting units, the responsible for the contracting and legal Intervention department, legal services and the contracting body.

For the development of the bidding process, at least the following steps should be developed:

1. Risk plan elaboration.
2. Approval of the procurement file and expenditure.
3. Preparation of the briefing of the Public Procurement of Innovation project specifications: governance model, contracts objectives, workplan, technical requirements and functional specifications, final choice of the type of Public Procurement of Innovation and preparation of the related standard specifications.
4. First bid alternatives document for each of the Public Procurement of Innovation projects.
5. First complete version of the PPI bidding documents.
6. Publication of the Public Procurement of Innovation bidding documents and evaluation of bids.

THE PUBLIC PROCUREMENT OF INNOVATION PROCESS: KEY STEPS

Award and Kick-Off

This process includes the award of the proposal, the presentation of the documentation by the contractor(s) and the execution of the contracts. In detail, it includes the following actions:

- Technical evaluation report with the results obtained in the evaluation process for the selected proposals.
- Management of claims, appeals and/or challenges to the process.
- Formalisation of the contract.

In this phase, a thorough planning of the Public Procurement of Innovation project should be conducted; its scope, the offer(s) received and a roadmap for an effective administrative, legal and technical follow-up should be established.

As a first step, a kick-off meeting should be organised with the parties involved to establish a governance structure for the Public Procurement of Innovation project and propose the roles, responsibilities and commitments of each of the parties; both on the part of the contracting body and on the part of the successful bidders. This initial Public Procurement of Innovation project kick-off meeting does not preclude the subsequent formalisation of the acceptance of each project plan at another meeting. The winning technical proposal(s) will be reviewed at these meetings.

Implementation of an Innovation Project

This involves all the administrative and document management tasks necessary to ensure the correct execution of the Public Procurement of Innovation project(s). The following methodology is proposed for each of the ongoing Public Procurement of Innovation projects:

- Preparation of the workplan with the key aspects: deadlines and milestones, presentation of the project schedule, indicators (KPIs), dedication of each of the components of the project team and establishment of the responsibility of each of them. Compliance with each requirement of the specifications should be monitored on an ongoing basis:
  - Verification that the task list is consistent with the objectives and scopes.
  - Verification that effort, costs, deadlines, equipment are consistent with the objectives and scopes.
- Management Plan (including methodology and data management).
- Risk Management Plan and Quality Assessment Plan.
- Detailed planning of documentation deliverables and deliverables resulting from the work, etc.

All this should be aligned with what was included in the bid and what was agreed in the planning of the PPI project.

Actions within the Public Procurement of Innovation Contracts

This process includes the development of a set of administrative actions related to the execution of the contract that may entail foreseen or unforeseen modifications, extensions, etc. during the execution of the contract.

A defined project management methodology must be put into practice to control the execution of the project and the follow-up of the work plan, focusing on the following aspects:

- Controls to ensure that the methodology and work plan are relevant to the stage the project is in, allowing for modifications when necessary.
- Controls for the quality of project deliverables and outcomes.
- Controls that ensure risks and deviations from the plan are assessed.
- Controls that actions and contingency measures are taken.

The monitoring and control of the tasks will be carried out, in addition to the deliverables required in each phase of the project, based on an interim report and a final phase report prepared by the awarded company(ies). This is a key aspect to ensure the correct project development and objectives. The company may be required to submit such reports as deemed necessary to determine whether:

- The company has used the resources foreseen and adequately carried out the activities planned for the phase it is executing (satisfactory completion).
- The project is progressing adequately towards the achievement of the final objectives (successful completion) and, therefore, the next phase has begun. For this purpose, the following must be prepared (if the tender is finally organised as a Commercial Public Procurement and in phases):
  - Information on recommendations, at the midpoint of the phase (if any), which allow the satisfactory or unsatisfactory fulfilment of the objectives of that phase, for payment purposes, as well as the passage to the next phase.
  - Final qualification information of phase results, which will allow the satisfactory or unsatisfactory fulfilment of the objectives of the first phase of this process to be determined for payment purposes, as well as the company or companies moving on to Phase 2 based on their successful completion.

The functional requirements, their phases, the milestones established for each phase and in the project planning and any changes to them that may be agreed upon by the parties through the procedures established for change management should be reviewed periodically, in accordance with the procedures established in the contract.

Technical and Administrative Closure of Public Procurement of Innovation Projects

This process includes checking the quality and volume of deliveries, to ensure their quality and consistency with the commitments set out in the awarding of each of the Public Procurement of Innovation contracts.

It is recommended that the results are reviewed based on the indicators established at the beginning and during the implementation of the project and following the procedures included in the Quality Assessment Plan. The information input channels for the review of the system of indicators and objectives are:

- The level of success of the objectives achieved.
- The evaluation of the processes.
- The evaluation of the organisation in relation to these activities.
- Evaluation by stakeholders (customers and collaborators).
- Assessment of the scalability of the developed product and evaluation of the road-to-market.

A good practice is to build a spreadsheet for each project properly prepared so that, as a report, it allows a quick and easy way to understand the tasks, deadlines and main indicators. In addition, it is advisable to hold a meeting per project to review the results obtained with a view to closing the project.

Deployment of the Results

In certain cases, the successful bidder will be expected to carry out detailed planning of the activities required from the end of the contract until the product reaches the market (subsequent validation studies, product compliance certification procedures, industrialisation activities, etc.).

The result of this phase is expected to be a complete product manual with its application protocols and expected performances, as well as the most suitable format for its use and a complete plan guiding its placing and market scalability.

Change Management

Change Management is identified as one of the main points of interest regarding the management and execution of Public Procurement of Innovation projects. To this end, models, methodologies, tools and procedure manuals should be articulated within the contracting administration to facilitate the incorporation of the new developments and procedures used during the execution of the service into the Administration's normal operations, to facilitate "learning for the future". Events to disseminate best practices, experience exchange and information about lessons learnt are highly recommended both within and external to the organisation.

FINAL REMARKS

Our understanding of a successful Innovation Procurement process is based on a good roadmap definition, where all the highlighted key steps that we have described are included. As an instrument to foster innovation, PPI should be understood in the context and strategic priorities of the region or country in which it will be developed in order to select the most adequate type of PPI. To achieve a successful PPI, it is mandatory from the outset to work in coordination with all the actors involved in the process, which will ensure a sufficient level of knowledge in the definition and development of all the stages described. As any other new strategy, to guarantee the future success of new initiatives, it is of great importance to develop information materials about the procedures and disseminate the results of successful projects, thus contributing to their progressive incorporation and PPI adoption.

REFERENCES

1. Public Procurement: OECD. https://www.oecd.org/gov/public-procurement/health/
2. Public Procurement: OECD. https://www.oecd.org/en/topics/public-procurement.html
3. EU Commission Guidance on Innovation Procurement. https://ec.europa.eu/docsroom/documents/45975
4. Public Procurement: OECD. https://www.oecd.org/en/topics/public-procurement.html
5. EU Commission: Shaping Europe's digital future (2022). https://wayback.archive-it.org/12090/20220916072752/https:/digital-strategy.ec.europa.eu/en/policies/pcp-and-pi-projects
6. Iqbal JD, Biller-Andorno N. The regulatory gap in digital health and alternative pathways to bridge it. *Health Policy and Technology*, 11 (3) 2022. https://doi.org/10.1016/j.hlpt.2022.100663
7. Manning CG. Technology Readiness Levels (2023). https://www.nasa.gov/directorates/somd/space-communications-navigation-program/technology-readiness-levels/
8. NextGenerationEU: For a stronger, more resilient Europe. https://next-generation-eu.europa.eu/index_es
9. European Regional Development Fund (EDRF). https://commission.europa.eu/funding-tenders/find-funding/eu-funding-programmes/european-regional-development-fund-erdf_en
10. EU Commission: Horizon Europe. https://commission.europa.eu/funding-tenders/find-funding/eu-funding-programmes/horizon-europe_en
11. European Health and Digital Executive Agency. https://hadea.ec.europa.eu/index_en
12. EU4Health: HaDEA. https://hadea.ec.europa.eu/programmes/eu4health/about_en
13. Interreg Europe. https://www.interregeurope.eu/

FURTHER READING

Procurement of ICT innovation. https://research-and-innovation.ec.europa.eu/strategy/support-policy-making/shaping-eu-research-and-innovation-policy/new-european-innovation-agenda/innovation-procurement_en

Public procurement as a driver of innovation in SMEs and public services. https://op.europa.eu/en/publication-detail/-/publication/f5fd4d90-a7ac-11e5-b528-01aa75ed71a1

3

Challenge Identification – How to Identify Innovation Needs?

Jorge González

INTRODUCTION

Do you have any idea how to start with a challenge identification? Start with pain points to address the problem in a better manner than the last time you did it. There is always an improved way to do everything, however you must think about this more than you did previously.

Understanding the importance of early identification of needs is crucial for a successful Innovation Procurement process. Innovation is key for addressing today and tomorrow's societal challenges. Innovation Procurement is one of the instruments to manage how innovation can be incorporated. By buying and implementing innovative solutions, healthcare service providers can have a positive impact on the quality of life of patients/citizens.

This chapter provides clues and processes that will help you when identifying unmet needs to trigger improvements within your organisation.

UNMET NEEDS IDENTIFICATION: WHAT AND WHO

The starting point for Innovation Procurement is "recognizing that you have an unmet need that requires a solution and then deciding to do something about it". [1]

Difference between a Need and a Solution

A need is the root problem you want to solve. A solution is the technology or approach to solve it. A need is something stable in time; for example, I want to move from point A to B as quickly and comfortably as possible. Solutions to this need include horses, bicycles, cars or airplanes.

When identifying and describing needs, try to isolate what is truly the problem, desire or outcome versus the technology that can solve it. First the need, then the solution. We strongly recommend focusing on describing the problem instead of how to solve it. Do not include the technology that can solve the problem when describing the need. For example, a good need description would never start with a sentence like "We need an app/blockchain/AI to do..."

Be aware of the risk of "technology fascination" when trying to adopt the latest cool technology to a problem. It may backfire if it is too costly for the problem at hand and you may overlook simpler or cheaper solutions that are easier to implement.

Therefore, put your efforts first on detecting pain points, inefficiencies or potential gains. Going through the description of the problem will give you the clues to think about the potential solutions that can be developed afterwards. Not investing enough time and brain power at this phase may have dire consequences later when you realise that the co-created solution is not really addressing the core problem, but rather the symptoms.

Difference between an Innovation Need and a Challenge

Needs and challenges are used imprecisely in common language. In this chapter, *a need* refers to the first draft of the identified pain point, inefficiency or potential gain. This is typically what the healthcare professional, manager or patient proposes with their own words and knowledge. However, this wording is not easy to be understood by potential solvers, requires further inputs from other organisational departments, for example, IT or legal, or lacks the right indicators to assess success at the end of the solution co-creation process.

We define *a challenge* as being when the work to "polish" the initial description of the need and improve it iteratively has been completed with the input and support from different stakeholders. The challenge is what will be shared with the supply side to recruit the best solver candidates.

Key Stakeholders to Be Involved in the Need Identification Process

More and more healthcare organisations depend on innovation units to support the identification of needs, matching with suppliers, looking for funding, co-creation of a solution, assessing results and promoting the adoption of the successful solution. Its support and experience are critical to manage an effective and efficient process through all phases. In case the organisation has no unit, at a very minimum, there must be a named person responsible for the initiative, ideally with supporting colleagues. It will be referred as the *Executive Team* within this document.

Healthcare professionals are at the front line of care and are a good source of needs and pain points to be solved. Not only can they identify these, but they are also critical in the solution-search process. In our jargon, the leading professional is called the "*intrapreneur*", that is, someone with an entrepreneurial spirit working within the healthcare organisation.

A very important role is that of the decision maker. Those with responsibility to make decisions on the importance of solving the need and, at the end of the process, allocate the resources to procure and implement must be incorporated at every step to maximise chances that the successfully developed solution has an impact on the patients, healthcare professionals and the organisation itself. Otherwise, there is a high risk of creating a successful solution to the need at hand and, then, nothing happens. The pilot does not survive the 'valley of death' and does not get implemented. All the effort and money are wasted. The innovation has no impact.

Finally, there may be other supporting services like IT, ethics, legal or other clinical colleagues that should be consulted and engaged during the refining of the initial unmet need description and, above all, during the development of a solution.

NEED IDENTIFICATION IN THE HEALTHCARE SECTOR: THE *INDEMAND* APPROACH

This section describes the methodology that Ticbiomed and its partners followed during the *inDemand* project: a demand-driven, co-creation model where Healthcare organisations and companies co-create Digital Health solutions, with the economic support of public regional funds. It is similar to other instruments like PCP or PPI, but leaner, faster and cheaper. Being demand-driven implies that the innovation finding approach starts with the identification of unmet needs.

The *inDemand* Model for Unmet Need Management

The methodological approach that was followed is described, from the preparation of the process (step 0) through to the assessment of its implementation (step 5).

STEP 0: Preparation of the Search for Needs

This step aims to prepare and launch a call for the needs of healthcare professionals and end-users. It sets up the documentation kit, guidelines, process and tools to select the best needs, considering the conditions and overall context of the healthcare organisation.

An Executive Team is set up to manage the whole process. The Team oversees defining the calendar, responsibilities and dissemination strategy. They also create the template for submission of unmet need proposals, set up the tools to collect them and develop the content for the open call dissemination.

For healthcare organisations that want to prioritise several strategic areas (*Topics*), a template was created to collect them. This information is used to highlight the Topics that are more relevant to the organisation and, therefore, have more chances to be selected for the follow-up steps. For the collection of needs (Step 2), a questionnaire was created. Its objective is to collect the unmet needs proposed by the intrapreneurs. An evaluation guideline was defined to be used by the Evaluation Committee in Step 3 to select the unmet needs that the organisation will promote their solution finding.

STEP 1: Recruitment

This phase aims to disseminate the call amongst the intrapreneurs to encourage the submission of high-quality proposals. It follows a dissemination plan. Also, it is important to create a contact list of those members of staff known for their entrepreneurial spirit.

A good dissemination campaign is critical to ensure that intrapreneurs fully understand the initiative, its process and the expected contribution from their side. Apart from the dissemination using corporate channels like emails and noticeboards, it is recommended to organise in-person events such as workshops to explain the initiative in more detail and solve questions.

STEP 2: Call for Needs

A call for needs is open for a limited time to collect the need proposals. Our recommendation is to publish an adapted version of the questionnaire into an online tool (e.g. Google forms) to have a unique point of collection of submissions.

The Executive Team should be available to deliver support and feedback to those potential applicants who ask for it.

STEP 3: Evaluation Committee and Final Decision

Step 3 aims to evaluate the submitted needs according to the eligibility and selection criteria previously defined. An Evaluation Committee is staffed with suitable experts/stakeholders that will review and select the most suitable proposals.

Each proposal is scanned to determine if it is eligible according to the rules of who and under what conditions a proposal can enter the process. This work is usually performed by the Execution Team.

Then, the Evaluation Committee proceeds to make the selection with reference to the Selection criteria. There is first an individual, asynchronous assessment by each committee member, that scores each proposal against the evaluation criteria. Each expert completes the evaluation template to record their scores.

The Execution Team then ranks the individual scores to produce a single list. For the top proposals, a collaborative assessment takes place in a meeting of the Evaluation Committee who jointly review them to develop a consensus score for each need. At the end of the meeting, the final ranking is established.

STEP 4: Communication of Results and Need Improvement

Once the needs have been selected the result is communicated to the applicants. It is important to manage disappointment effectively for those not awarded to encourage intrapreneurs to participate in future iterations. For those selected, the Execution Team supports them to develop the submitted need into a challenge. Organisation information like technical, legal, ethical, data protection and corporate standards for exchanging information are incorporated into the initial description. Very importantly, a refinement of the indicators that will be used to confirm if the solution provides the expected results at the end of its development takes place.

If finding an effective solution for the unmet need is anticipated to be done in collaboration with an external company, it is recommended that market-related information like the size of expected population to benefit from the solution is acquired.

The examples below may help understand how initial submissions become much more informative and impactful after these inputs are incorporated. The polishing of the need is an iterative process that requires the input and validation of several stakeholders. The final version of the challenge should be reviewed and approved by the decision makers (*e.g.* Top management) before moving to the next phase in the Innovation Procurement process; typically, the search for an external company to co-create the solution or the establishment of an internal team to develop the solution internally.

Figure 3.1 The inDemand stepwise process

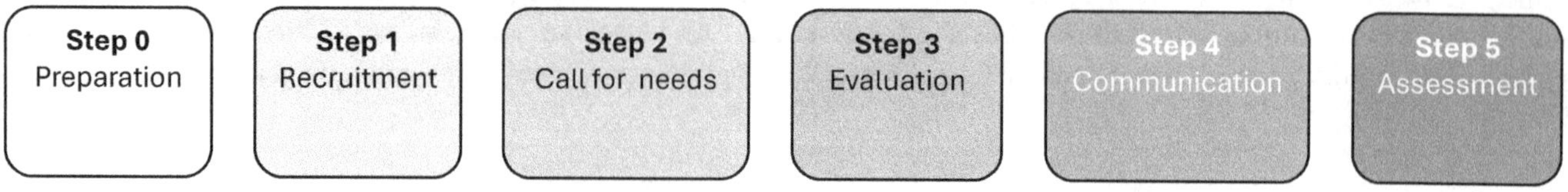

Figure 3.2 Actions required for the search for needs

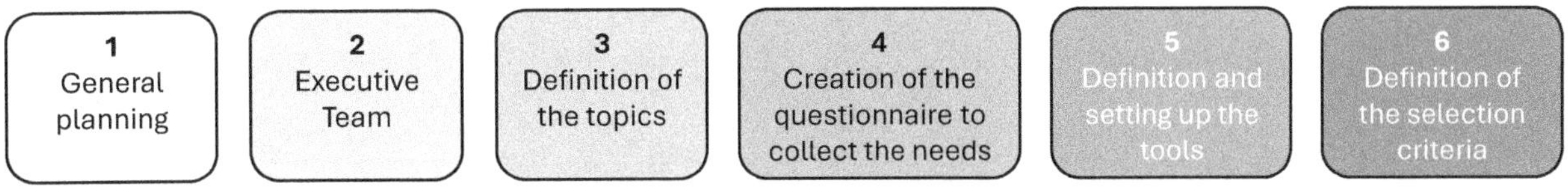

Figure 3.3 Actions required for recruitment of intrapreneurs

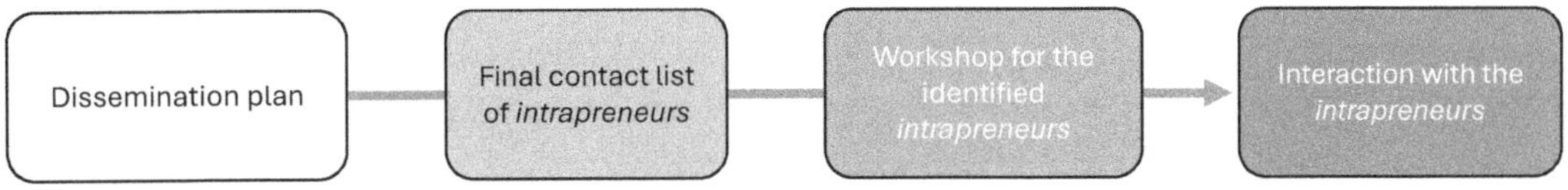

STEP 5: Assessment

This final step collects and reviews the issues, lessons learnt and best practices. It then proposes and documents improvements for the next iteration. This is especially valuable for the Execution Teams to become expert in the model execution over time and, therefore, help to generate a positive culture towards innovation in the organisation.

Key Considerations from the Different Stages

In the previous section, we have considered briefly the different phases for the needs' identification within a healthcare organisation and key documents you may find helpful to proceed are available in the resources at the end of the chapter, so that you can have useful examples for your need identification process, if needed. Nevertheless, we do not want to conclude this section without highlighting critical aspects you should bear in mind in each of the stages when identifying unmet needs. These are set out in table 3.1.

PRACTICAL EXAMPLES FROM THE *INDEMAND* PROJECT

Four challenges were selected in Murcia Region of Spain within the *inDemand* project:

Challenge 1: ACRA (Avoiding Care Re-Admission).
Challenge 2: MENUDO (Child obesity support solution for healthcare providers and families).
Challenge 3: EPITIC (Digital patient-doctor communication channel for epilepsy management).
Challenge 4: HEAT (HEAlthcare Training management platform).

EPITIC "Digital Patient-Doctor Communication Channel for Epilepsy Management"

Challenge 3 (EPITIC) is described in more detail as a practical example from the *inDemand* project.

Pitch

A solution that leverages existing corporate IT systems to facilitate the empowerment of patients with epilepsy, and their convenient communication with doctors.

Main Objective

The main objective of this challenge is to improve the quality of life experienced by patients with epilepsy by facilitating a more convenient communication with the doctor and helping them to better manage their condition. As a secondary objective, the challenger also wants to learn how to easily integrate third party patient facing mobile solutions with its corporate IT systems.

Figure 3.4 Actions required the call for needs

Figure 3.5 Actions required for the Evaluation committee

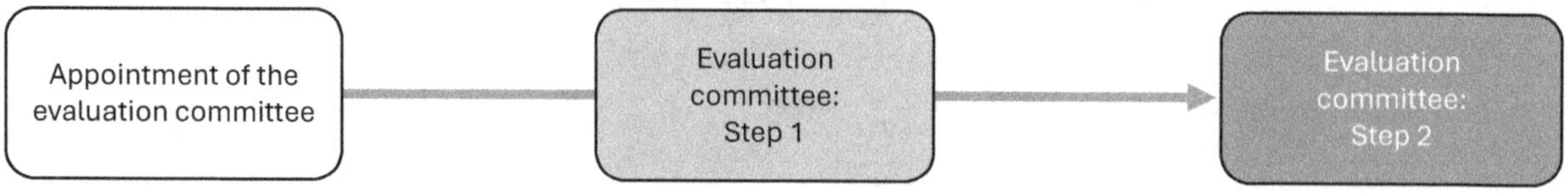

Pilot Functional Scope

Compulsory Requirements

- Information exchange channel between patients and doctors (neurologists).
- Patients would choose from several templates to create the message, depending on the message type.
- Doctors should be able to send the same message to different patient groupings.
- The records of exchanges should be accessible any time.
- Calendar management. So, patients and doctors can easily add and review historical data about epileptic episodes.
- Alert doctors that a relevant event or incidence needs their attention. Ideally configurable by their channel(s) of preference (email, alert in smart phone, electronic health record, etc).
- Facilitate access to informative resources for self-empowerment, like documents and videos. Including a survey to assess the QUOLIE-10 indicator [3] and a mechanism to request and collect the patient outcomes over time.
- It must be usable and intuitive, especially for patients.

Desirable Requirements

- Medication management. Possibility that doctors incorporate and modify prescriptions.
- Ideally integrated with Servicio Murciano Salud (SMS) corporate medication system.
- Supporting added value tools, like reminders and/or patient adherence encouragement via gamification.
- Connection with third party devices like smart bands to track sleep patterns and/or exercise.
- Information summaries and analytics on the available data to empower patients and facilitate better disease management by the patients themselves, in collaboration with their doctors.
- Optimised for multi-device access (desktop, mobile device, etc.) for doctors and patients.

Pilot Set-Up (Requirements and Compliance)

After a selection process conducted by the challenger, 30 patients enrolled in the pilot together with three neurologists.

Ethical and Data Protection

The pilot methodology must be approved by an Ethics Committee of the SMS. The Committee will pay special attention to the collection of informed consent of patients by solver and the protection of personal data, observing the requirements established by the new European Data Protection Regulation and the Spanish law. Among other requirements, an Impact Analysis with identified risks and proposed measures will be required from the Solver.

If deemed necessary, the Solver will be asked to anonymise the data according to mechanisms established by the Challenger. At any case, the Solver cannot exploit or make use of the data for different purposes than the ones agreed with the Challenger, and after pilot end, all copies of the data must be transferred back to the Challenger or deleted.

Figure 3.6 Actions required during assessment

Table 3.1 Key considerations at the different stages

STEP	CONSIDERATIONS
Step 0	Topics should be selected by senior management, based on organisational strategy
Step 1	Very important personal connections to make aware and engage participants. Contact key opinion leaders to multiply and motivate
Step 2	Continuous interaction and feedback with the intrapreneurs will increase the quantity and quality of the proposal
Step 3	Carefully identify and staff the evaluation committee. Block out their diaries in advance, as they tend to be saturated
Step 4	Look for alternatives of support for those that have not been selected
Step 5	Document the improvements, so that the know-how is passed on, even if members of the Executive Team are not available for the next iteration

Technological

When the pilot starts there will be an App available for local patients developed by the SMS that incorporates, among others, user authentication. The new App developed by the Solver must be called from the SMS App, so user identification takes place leveraging corporate mechanisms via the OAuth standard. The Solver App will notify the SMS systems about certain events and situations. Ideally via HL7 messaging, but web services could be an option. This information may include registration status, activity, progress and periodic (summarised) clinical information. The systems and servers needed for running the piloted App will be hosted by the Solver. If the complexity of the connections is too high or the personal data could be at risk, these systems should be hosted in SMS servers. This will be established in a technical session at the beginning of the project. In any event the Solver will provide mechanisms to guarantee that SMS can exploit the data. The solver App will be available for Android and iOS.

Data

No initial data will be provided for pre-load. All participants will have to register for free and fill their own data.

Expected Impact and KPIs

- QUOLIE-10 indicator. Increase of an average of 2.5 points per month of usage, with a maximum of 10 points during the total intervention period.
- Reduction in number of epileptic crises in patients. Equivalent to 20% in a whole year, based on intervention duration.
- Reduction in the number of physical visits of patients: (A) To the doctor office: at least by 15% for the medium of the group of patients involved and (B) To the emergency room: at least by 20%.
- The SMS will study the possibility of developing an analysis of the economic impact by the methodology of Social Return of Investment (SROI) to make the decision for scaling-up this solution.

Business Opportunity

At the level of the SMS, this project would be replicable in nine Neurology services, with around 50 neurologists apart from training specialists (resident doctors). At national level, there are 30–50 epilepsy related units in public hospitals, with at least 700 neurologists working in them. Potential users are estimated in 8,700 patients in the Region of Murcia and 278,400 in Spain.

This communication channel can be extended in a standard way with the same technology to many other pathologies, inside and outside SMS, with a great possibility of growth.

Lessons Learnt from the *inDemand* Project

After a long identification of unmet needs process within the *inDemand* project, several lessons learnt and recommendations to improve the process were identified.

Preparation of the Search for Needs

- The involvement of all actors is key. Intrapreneurs must be aware of the process that is being implemented so they are motivated to participate in development at later stages of the co-creation process.
- The selection of services areas aligned with the hospital strategy is a critical part of the preparation of the search for needs. It is also recommended that the key experts and the management responsible for those services will be involved in the process from the very beginning.
- The definition of topics is a powerful tool as it facilitates the alignment with the priorities of the top management at the healthcare organisation.
- To facilitate the scoring during the evaluation process, the questionnaire must be fully aligned with the selection criteria.

Launch of the Search of Needs

- To involve the stakeholders and disseminate the content of the Call for needs, a summary document presenting the co-creation model is needed.
- Incentives to the intrapreneurs (not financial because they work by internal motivation, but about visibility and recognition) are highly recommended. As a clear example, the General Manager from Servicio Murciano de Salud issued a signed certificate for each proposal, winner or not, just for the effort, as a sign of merit for their professional career.
- Prior to the Call for needs launch the organisation of a Workshop is key to ensure a good understanding of the model from potential Intrapreneurs and develop interest and motivation from the hospital's personal to be involve in the project.
- A methodology on how to define an unmet need for the Intrapreneurs is really helpful. Healthcare professionals can find it difficult to describe the current problems they are facing and translate them into a need that can be understood and addressed by solvers.

Evaluation and Selection of Needs

- To choose the most suitable needs, the evaluation must be conducted in two phases. The first phase of the assessment will be handled by the innovation staff/innovation experts, the hospital managers responsible for the services to be dealt with and the key experts of the presented needs. In the second phase, the sufficient management seniority level of the hospital will make the final decisions.
- Different documents are required for the process: the Call for needs questionnaire filled by Challengers and the challenges document published by Funder for the Call for Solvers. The first one outlines the needs while the second collects technical requirements without clinical comments. A "translation" work is necessary after the selection of the need and before the Call for Solvers to get a polished document to be launched for the call.
- Once the challenges are collected, they must be transferred to Funder in the local language. The Funder may otherwise source translation from external agency who is not familiar with healthcare, and this can result in the use of strange terms and non-healthcare vocabulary in the call for solutions.
- Take enough time to support and screen all proposals. Give more time to write, help and support for assessment, screening and final evaluation.

OTHER PROJECTS REPLICATING THE *INDEMAND* MODEL

Ticbiomed has a wide experience on identification of unmet needs within healthcare organisations. For that reason, we can include other good examples that have replicated the *inDemand* model for the identification of unmet needs.

InnoBuyer [4]

InnoBuyer implements a demand-driven methodology that brings together Challengers (public and private organisations) and Solvers (notably European Innovation Council-supported SMEs), to jointly co-create innovative solutions, and speed up the process leading to the procurement of such innovation. InnoBuyer provides financial support to Challengers and Suppliers in 4 actions:

- **Action 1: Recruitment and aggregation of Challengers**
  The InnoBuyer consortium has launched a dissemination campaign to recruit unmet needs from Challengers and the 15 best candidates have been selected.
- **Action 2: Buyer-SME matching**
  The selected Challengers will be supported to launch an Open Market Consultation to receive feedback on their challenges, and recruit and award Solvers to answer the proposed challenges.
- **Action 3: Pilot co-creation**
  Challengers and Solvers will jointly co-create solutions to the challenges. The solutions will be tested and evaluated. Solvers will receive support towards the future commercialisation of their solutions.
- **Action 4: Legal support to launch a tender**
  If the co-creation results are successful, Challenger will receive support for the creation of the terms of reference in collaboration with external experts, as the base for a future procurement for the solution by the Challengers.

InnoBuyer is an optimised version of the *inDemand* model. While *inDemand* model was implemented within the healthcare organisation only, InnoBuyer is applicable to external organisation outside the project consortium.

HealthChain [5]

HealthChain aims to create demand-driven Digital Health solutions by fostering collaboration between Healthcare Organisations (HOs) and IT companies. With a focus on co-creation and adoption, HealthChain brings together a diverse consortium of eighteen partners spanning five regional ecosystems across different EU countries, ensuring a holistic and inclusive approach to transforming healthcare.

Ticbiomed is driving the efforts of the HealthChain consortium that it is strategically designed to encompass the regional ecosystems of Murcia (Spain), Centro (Portugal), Western (Slovenia), Primorsko-Goranska (Croatia), and East Netherlands (Netherlands). Each region plays a vital role, with HOs identifying challenges and piloting proposed solutions, two IT companies (Solvers) collaborating to develop these solutions, and a regional Ecosystem Supporter (ES) facilitating cross-border connections among regions.

Cherries [6]

Cherries aimed at enabling Responsible, Research and Innovation (RRI) policy experiments in the healthcare sector in three European territories: Murcia (ES), Örebro (SE) and the Republic of Cyprus (CY). The Cherries team applies the RRI framework to mobilise territorial stakeholder ecosystems and engage them in regional pilot actions aimed at:

1. Identifying needs in the healthcare sector at the territorial level.
2. Encourage the proposition and co-creation of innovative solutions to the identified needs.
3. Stimulate institutional reflection processes on innovating products and services in the healthcare sector through participatory approaches.
4. Present evidence-based recommendations for revising sectoral policies, strategies and innovation support instruments.

inDemand RCT [7]

InDemand-RCT, entails performing a Randomised Control Trial (RCT) to check the efficacy of an innovation support model for SMEs (*inDemand* model, innovation driven by demand). It was put into effect to meet the innovation, digitalisation and Covid-19 response needs identified by large/tractor companies in the Region of Murcia (Spain). The technological challenges identified by large/tractor companies were from economic sectors included in the Smart Specialisation Strategy of the Murcia region.

The main objective of the project was to compare the *inDemand* model with Business Co-Creation and Support with the *inDemand* method without these support services. Taking into account the differential characteristics, the *inDemand* model with co-creation and business support is expected to be more successful than the standalone *inDemand* model.

CLOSING REMARKS

The identification of unmet needs within the healthcare organisations is a complex process where all stakeholders must be involved from the very beginning. Engaging intrapreneurs and end-users to take part in the identification of unmet needs is key to getting a successful challenge defined to co-create a solution that cover and satisfy such an unmet need.

In recent years, several projects have been launched to establish common methodologies to be followed by the healthcare organisations from different EU countries. Ticbiomed are fully committed to improve the process after each project by identifying key lessons learnt so that they can be incorporated in the next project we are involved in.

From our experience, each project has their own peculiarities, and a solution cannot always be adopted due to the complexity of Public Procurement of Innovation in the healthcare sector. This is why we want to move forward to get faster, leaner and more cost-effective instruments and increase the chances that innovative solutions are adopted after successful pilots. A win-win approach is key to motivate all stakeholders involved, given that they are putting all their efforts into it, and they expect to advance and obtain benefits instead of wasting their time and money.

RESOURCES

The documents referred in the *inDemand* project have been included for a better understanding of the methodology for the identification of unmet needs process. These are key templates that you can replicate to identify unmet needs within your own organisation.

Definition of topics: https://procure4health.eu/wp-content/uploads/2023/08/P4H_Insight-3_inDemand-Annex-1.pdf

Call for challenges questionnaire: https://procure4health.eu/wp-content/uploads/2023/08/P4H_Insight-3_inDemand-Annex-2.pdf

Evaluation committee and criteria: https://procure4health.eu/wp-content/uploads/2023/08/P4H_Insight-3_inDemand-Annex-3.pdf

Annex 4: Evaluation Template: https://procure4health.eu/wp-content/uploads/2023/08/P4H_Insight-3_inDemand-Annex-4.pdf

Annex 5: Template challenges to funders: https://procure4health.eu/wp-content/uploads/2023/08/P4H_Insight-3_inDemand-Annex-5.pdf

REFERENCES

1. Whyles G. BIS Consultant FCP Programme Manager (JERA Consulting). *Personal communication.*
2. In Demand. https://www.indemandhealth.eu/
3. Viteri C, Codina M, Cobaleda S, Lahuerta J, Barriga J, Barrera S, Morales MD; grupo de investigadores del estudio de validación del cuestionario QOLIE-10. Validación de la versión española del cuestionario de calidad de vida en epilepsia QOLIE-10 [Validation of the Spanish version of the QOLIE-10 quality of life in epilepsy questionnaire]. *Neurologia.* 2008 Apr;23(3):157-167. https://pubmed.ncbi.nlm.nih.gov/18370335/- PubMed.
4. Innobuyer: Fast track to Innovation Procurement. https://innobuyer.eu/innobuyer-call -for-challengers-winners/
5. Healthchain. https://healthchain-i3.eu/
6. Cherries: Responsible healthcare ecosystems. https://www.cherries2020.eu/
7. Info. https://www.institutofomentomurcia.es/indemand-rct-open-call-murcia-2021

4

Ten Things You Need to Consider When Preparing Your Innovation Tender

Ana Lucia Jaramillo Villacís and Beatriz Gómez Fariñas

INTRODUCTION

Public procurement is an important driver for the green and digital transformation of the public sector. It represents around 14% of GDP in the EU and helps create an economy that is more innovative and socially inclusive, improving the quality and efficiency of public services.

Innovation Procurement is an important tool at the disposal of policymakers to solve important societal challenges that Europe is facing in various key sectors, including health care. Innovation Procurement happens when public buyers acquire the development or deployment of pioneering innovative solutions to address specific mid-to-long-term public-sector needs. This approach fosters innovation from the demand side and helps shape markets as well as create new ones, thus creating opportunities for small and medium enterprises (SMEs).

Although Innovation Procurement entails important benefits in terms of adequacy of the solution, modernisation of the public services and efficient use of the public funds, it is not unusual that public buyers are reluctant to apply it due to the lack of knowledge and expertise on how to conduct such a procurement. In this chapter, we set out 10 key aspects to prepare your Innovation Procurement project successfully. From the identification of your needs to the publication of the tender, the step-by-step approach explained below provides all the information you need to start thinking about the actions to be carried out and the necessary resources

Innovation Procurement includes:

- The development of innovative solutions through the procurement of Research and Development (R&D) services. This is possible by conducting a Pre-Commercial Procurement (PCP).
- The procurement of innovative solutions that are not yet available or do not exist on the market; or the procurement of innovative solutions that do exist but are not yet widely available on the market. In this case, the public buyer acts as a launch customer through Public Procurement of Innovative Solutions (PPIs).

The preparation of the contract is essential in any public procurement procedure to ensure the feasibility of the contract, the full satisfaction of the public buyer's needs and an efficient spending of the public funds. Increasingly, society demands the acquisition of better products and services at a lower price, and to achieve this result, it is essential that the contract is properly designed and followed by the conduct of a modern and efficient procurement procedure. In the case of PPI, this phase takes on special relevance, as this modality requires strategic planning in the light of the public buyer's medium and long-term objectives.

The design and preparation of the contract is key for the success of your Innovation Procurement project, and therefore you should allocate special attention and effort at this stage. In the next pages, you will get a clear picture of 10 strategic aspects to take into consideration when preparing an innovation tender.

1. WORK IN A STRUCTURED WAY

If you are considering initiating an Innovation Procurement project, the first step is to become familiar with how it works and embrace a solid methodology that allows you to assess the feasibility of the project.

A fantastic example of a solid and comprehensive methodology is the approach developed under the European Assistance For Innovation Procurement (EAFIP) initiative of the European Commission. This initiative supports public procurers across Europe in developing and implementing Innovation Procurement, promoting good practices and encouraging them to use this instrument to boost the digital-green economy recovery.

The EAFIP step-by-step methodology is based upon the Plan, Do, Check, Act (PDCA) approach. First, you must understand the problems/needs that you have in your organisation and plan potential solutions to solve them, for example, by purchasing innovative solutions. It is advised to compile your needs in the short and medium term in a demand plan to easily assess which of them should be satisfied first, on the one hand, and inform the technology vendors about your needs so they are aware of them and plan accordingly, on the other.

Once you have a well-defined need that you intend to satisfy through Innovation Procurement, the next step is to explore whether this approach is suitable, and under which conditions, by exploring what the market can offer, engaging with technology vendors and conducting a cost-benefit analysis. If this assessment shows that there are no solutions available in the market to fully cover your needs and the project is economically feasible, then it is possible to conduct an Innovation Procurement process.

The next step is to prepare and publish the tender, followed by the award and execution of the contract(s).

2. HAVE A CLEAR PICTURE OF WHAT YOU NEED

The Innovation Procurement process starts with an unmet need for innovation solution, that is, a need that cannot be satisfied with the products or services already available in the market or can only be satisfied at excessive cost or with unacceptable risk.

It is essential for public buyers to identify unmet needs within their organisation on a regular basis to:

1. Have sufficient time for an effective understanding of the needs.
2. Develop a plan to ensure their timely satisfaction.
3. Avoid unidentified needs becoming an urgent problem.

Once the needs have been identified, it is time to decide which of them should be satisfied in the short, medium, or long term.

You should capture your needs in a clear and simple manner, focusing on describing the problem and the required functionalities rather than prescribing a specific solution. This approach allows the market to be creative and propose the most adequate solution for your problem (within the budget and timeframe described in the tender).

EXAMPLE – TECHNOLOGY NEUTRAL NEEDS A DESCRIPTION

A requirement for "electric vehicles" sounds innovative, but the technology neutral requirement is more likely to be a "low carbon zero emission vehicle" (to give equal chances to solutions based on other technological approaches to compete on the market).

See Department for Business Innovation & Skills, "Delivering best value through innovation. Forward Commitment Procurement. Practical Pathways to Buying Innovative Solutions", November 2011, available at:

https://www.gov.uk/government/uploads/system/uploads/attachment_data/file/32446/11-1054-forward-commitment-procurement-buying-innovative-solutions.pdf.

3. INVOLVE PRACTITIONERS AND END-USERS IN THE DEFINITION OF THE NEEDS

When defining the functionalities of the desired solution, it is essential to consider the point of view of practitioners and end-users, since usually they are in a better position to understand the problem and define the aspects that need to be solved. It is important to keep in mind that Innovation Procurement needs to be driven by their needs, otherwise the innovative solutions coming out of the procurement will not be accepted and/or used afterwards. If your organisation is not an end-user, it is recommended to involve the real end-users in this process.

To do so, as a starting point, you can organise meetings or informal chats within your organisation. It is essential to involve the management team in the discussions to ensure that you will receive the support and financial resources for the procurement. The discussions can be structured in focus groups which target, for example, different types of activities or policy objectives, and could include the participation of external experts and/or key stakeholders along with the public procurer's representatives. If needed, this can be complemented with surveys to end-users conducted by email, phone or post.

EXAMPLE – IDENTIFYING AND ASSESSING THE END-USER NEEDS

SMART@FIRE PCP PROJECT

The EU funded Smart@Fire PCP project considered that it was important to:

- Identify and understand the real needs of the end-users (in this case, fire-fighters, the intervention coordination officers, medical and physical trainers, maintenance crews, etc.).
- Formulate these needs in functional terms.
- To ensure that the needs identified by the procurers in the Smart@Fire project (FR and BE procurers) were aligned with the needs of fire brigades all across Europe, in total, 961 fire brigades from 16 EU countries were involved in the needs identification and assessment exercise.
- The **needs identification** exercise was based on the following main question: "*How to increase the safety and reduce risks of first responders undertaking fire-fighting and other civil protection work?*"
- The needs identification was conducted through a large-scale survey, face-to-face needs assessment meetings and interviews. To contextualise the needs identification into the real working environment, short scenarios (use-cases) were outlined. These **use-cases** sketched a contextual situation with significant details, allowing a fire-fighter to unambiguously imagine the circumstances and assess the conditions. A good scenario comprises multiple elements. The subject of the scenario is mostly the specific end-user (in this case, the fire-fighter).
- There is also an action involved (e.g. falling down), as well as a positive conclusion of the scenario provided by the added value of a new feature or product (e.g. the fall detection sensor and signal, heartbeat sensor, oxygen level sensor). The list of use-cases is typically constructed via interviews with selected relevant and-users.
- The following stage of **needs assessment** consisted of several interviews with selected relevant end-users to validate whether a certain need is correctly interpreted, expressed, assessed and valued in terms of importance for the fire-fighters. The relevant end-users were selected based on a pre-defined profile.
- The needs assessment exercise showed that the following features of a smart Personal Protective Systems (PPS) are highly desirable for the surveyed fire-fighters:
- A **localisation** of the firefighter and their team, in buildings and open areas, displayed on a map, made available to the firefighter and the intervention coordinating officer.
- **Remote parameter monitoring and historical logging**, making the info accessible via an intuitive dashboard for the officer (e.g. a map), enriched with the status of the team, their PPS, and the environment, enabling threshold setting and generating (automatic) alerts.
- Monitoring the environment, more in particular **temperature, temperature evolution, hotspot detection and presence of explosive gasses**.
- General requirements as robustness under mechanical friction, maintenance, repair, cleaning, with easy mounting/dismounting of the ICT and ideally with self-assessment.
- This exercise motivated the decision of Smart@fire to focus the scope of the PCP on the localisation challenge that was shared and ranked as highly important by all surveyed fire-fighters.
- For more information, see: https://cordis.europa.eu/article/id/190725-how-better-pcp-could-save-firefighters-lives

4. UNDERSTAND WHAT THE MARKET CAN OFFER

Once you have defined your need in a functional way, the next step is to conduct a state-of-the-art analysis to identify what is available in the market and the Technology Readiness Level (TRL) of the solutions. It gathers all relevant information available in the public domain (existing products, product under development, published literature and scientific studies) whether IPR protected or not. To do so, it is essential to ensure that the individual or team responsible for the search has relevant technological, industry and scientific expertise. In addition, this exercise may be complemented with conversation with experts in the relevant market such as research institutions, retailers, buyers or other people associated with the creation of innovative technologies.

If the market analysis reveals that solutions are already available on the market that can meet your needs or will become available before the end of the planned procurement, then there is no need for an Innovation Procurement and an existing solution can be procured. When purchasing solutions, you may want to assess, on a case-by-case basis, the convenience of inserting value engineering clauses in the contract to incentive suppliers to come up with innovations and lower the Total Cost of Ownership (TCO) along the term of the contract.

5. INTERACT WITH THE MARKET

Conducting a EU-wide market consultation, which should be announced in the Tenders Electronic Daily (TED) through a Prior Information Notice (PIN), will provide the necessary basis for starting the procurement.

The market consultation is important in several ways:

It enables you to cross-check the market analysis previously performed and helps validate the innovation potential of the need:

1. It provides feedback on how to raise interest from the market to answer to the upcoming call for tender, the type of players on the market and what they can offer.
2. It makes potential interested bidders aware of the public procurers' needs.
3. It allows cross-checking of the feasibility and market acceptance of the envisaged contract set-up (key contractual conditions, budget, timeframe, etc.).

To achieve these objectives, there are some aspects that you need to consider:

1. Communicate the identified needs openly and clearly to all potentially interested bidders (including the costs of the existing solution and the results of the market analysis).
2. Mention your desire for an innovative outcome in the announcement of the market consultation.
3. Give the suppliers sufficient time to ask questions and provide their views on the progress of ongoing product development and the feasibility of the proposed procurement approach.
4. Identify the right market segments and effectively disseminate the market consultation well in advance to ensure broad participation.
5. Guarantee the security of confidential information, trade secrets and intellectual property.

EXAMPLE – OPEN MARKET CONSULTATION: PRO-LITE PROJECT

In 2014, Transport for London (TfL) started Open Market Consultations to get feedback from the market about its plans to deploy more energy-efficient lighting systems for the London underground system. This exercise was conducted in the context of the EU-funded PPI project PRO-LITE, which aimed at driving competition and stimulating innovation within the lighting market across Europe.

The Open Market Consultation included presenting at Europe's largest lighting conferences, as well as the development and use of online submission tools, including questionnaires, through which manufacturers and suppliers were able to outline information on their organisation's capabilities, innovative technologies, and their experiences working with others to innovate. Furthermore, in mid-2015 TfL hosted a "Suppliers Morning" event to engage with potential suppliers of lighting innovation face to face. TfL invited over 60 lighting manufacturers and suppliers that responded to their market engagement e-Form, as well as representatives from Europe's Lighting Industry Association who helped the organisation to acquire information on almost 300 innovative lighting technologies.

Due to the wide-ranging method used to organise the market engagement exercise, PRO-LITE partners have engaged over 100 lighting manufacturers and suppliers at lighting conferences and other events and received written information from organisations based in over 10 countries from across Europe, North America and Asia.

The expertise gathered during the Open Market Consultation was used to inform the procurement processes employed during and beyond the PRO-LITE project life-cycle; namely to develop the performance requirements, the technical specifications and the procurement documents.

Source: https://procuraplus.org/fileadmin/user_upload/Activities_files/Events/Webinar_Award_Winners/Leon_Smith_TfL.pdf

6. GET A CLEAR PICTURE OF THE COSTS, BENEFITS AND VALUE OF YOUR PROJECT

Develop a business case based on a cost/benefit analysis of the solutions you aim to purchase to fulfil your need. The analysis of the costs versus benefits of starting an Innovation Procurement is conducted for each unmet need defined in terms of functionality/performance improvements, for which no solutions are available in the market [2].

The "business case" provides the economic justification (cost benefit analysis) to decide for which unmet needs it makes most sense to start an Innovation Procurement. It enables the procurer to prioritise unmet needs according to their highest potential impact versus costs. The business case also provides insights on how to practically organise the procurement to maximise expected impacts, whilst keeping the costs and risks to an acceptable level.

The business case establishes:

- What should be the maximum budget and duration for the procurement to keep costs to an acceptable proportion of the expected benefits.
- The minimum number of vendors to be engaged to reduce the risk that nobody can deliver a working solution.
- How to set the "minimum" functionality/performance requirements to achieve the minimum quality/efficiency improvements needed.
- What are the benefits/drawbacks to split the procurement into lots and what are the dependencies between different lots.
- Which test set-up is most suitable to check whether expected impacts are reached or not etc.

The business case also enables the procurer to perform a sensitivity analysis on each of the key project management parameters to quantify upfront what the positive/negative impact will be if one of these parameters changes during the project (worst-/best-case analysis). During the Open Market Consultation, you can verify the setting of the project the "sensitivity to change" (to understand whether the assumptions of the business case were realistic or not). If needed, you can modify the business case/the parameter settings for the procurement.

You can use the business case as a tool to support investment and project management decisions before, during and after the project:

1. **Before the project:** To determine whether there is enough economic justification to start the procurement and to set key parameters for organising the procurement set-up in such a way to maximise expected impacts, whilst keeping the costs and risks to an acceptable predefined level.
2. **During the project:** To decide how to best monitor vendors' performance and to project-manage the procurement to balance costs and benefits; to decide how to best deal with unexpected events inside the project or changes in the environment around the project.
3. **After the project:** To assess whether the results achieved meet the public procurer's goals (based on expected impacts defined initially in the business case before starting the project); to draw lessons learned and better prepare future procurements (e.g. to prepare a PPI after a PCP).

During a PCP or PPI project, the business case is the main control tool that is referenced on a regular basis by the project manager to ensure that the project remains viable. The cost/benefit analysis of a business case for starting a project is based on three financial indicators: the Net Present Value (NPV), the Internal Rate of Return (IRR) and the Return On Investment (ROI).

- The NPV is used to assess the overall profitability of a project, at the time when the public procurer needs to decide whether to start a project.
- The IRR is related to NPV and represents the interest rate for which the NPV of the project is equal to zero, that is NPV = 0, namely, the rate at which the costs of the project equalise its benefits, and profit margin is zero.
- The last important financial indicator to compute is ROI, defined as the NPV of a project divided by the investments made.

Typically, the procurer of an Innovation Procurement project would expect the business case to demonstrate a positive NPV, reflecting the value created after accounting for the time value of money, usually benchmarked against a discount rate like the bank interest rate. While ROI can offer a simple performance indicator, it should not be directly compared with interest rates unless it is time-adjusted. From a purely economic perspective, a project with a positive NPV should be considered for progression, even if its static ROI is lower than the bank interest rate.

Financial viability is typically not the only consideration for a public procurer to consider when deciding whether to start an Innovation Procurement. A public procurer also may need to include broader policy considerations such as environmental and social aspects in the business case. If the benefits of those broader policy considerations (the added value of the project) cannot be fully quantified financially and brought into the business case computation; this may justify undertaking the project even when NPV < 0. Likewise, still for policy-related reasons, a public procurer may decide not to start an Innovation Procurement project even NPV > 0. For example, an Innovation Procurement may be able to generate a 5% cost reduction over four years, but this may not be enough to start a financially demanding project.

7. BE CLEAR HOW YOU WANT TO PROCURE

Design your procurement strategy, including the choice of procedure and the provisions to include in the tender documents, based on the analysis of the results of your market consultation and business case.

A procurement strategy is a long-term plan to ensure a smooth procurement process to purchase the specified solutions accurately, punctually and in a cost-effective manner with good risk management. A clear procurement strategic plan can support your organisation to achieve its goals and avoids ambiguity for suppliers. It also helps set objectives and measure the effectiveness of procurement against the goals.

Ideally, a procurement strategy should reduce the Total Cost of Ownership (TCO), while also ensuring high quality and timely supplies and mitigating risks. Risk mitigation is an important function of procurement. When certain supplies are critical to production, any unforeseen disruption in their supply could disrupt the entire supply chain. Therefore, assessing the potential risk factors should form part of supplier selection.

In Innovation Procurement, the procurement strategy will be defined based on the maturity of the solutions that could address the unmet need. The maturity of the solutions is assessed based on the Technology Readiness Levels (TRL: see Number 4 above).

8. SET UP MECHANISMS TO MONITOR THE CONTRACT EXECUTION

Establish contract monitoring milestones and KPIs that can be monitored and assessed to improve. Prepare upfront the ways in which you will evaluate the project and, after its completion, extract and share lessons learned. Monitoring involves continuous follow-up during the execution of the Innovation Procurement project and entails the evaluation of performance with regards to the planned objectives, results, activities and means. To monitor how the contract is executed it is important to collect and evaluate performance data and provide appropriate feedback.

Effective and continuous oversight will prevent poor performance by the economic operator and will ensure proper expenditure of the public money. To be able to monitor the performance of the economic operator, the public procurer should begin by creating a list of the performance indicators ("*SMART indicators*" or "*Key Performance Indicators (KPIs)*"), against which the activity of the economic operator will be judged. The SMART indicators or KPIs are a type of measurement of the economic operator's success in achieving certain levels of operational goals, for example, no defects in a product or customer satisfaction, or progress toward strategic goals.

In addition, intermediate targets (*milestones*) for the achievement of a specific objective will express the progress set for the end of a period, which is shorter than the contract term. The economic operator will be required to identify in its proposal suitable milestones for the performance framework. These milestones are assessed during the initial tender evaluation and are subsequently used to monitor the contract.

In general terms, monitoring and assessment systems use different types of indicators:

1. **Quantitative indicators:** Are statistical measures of results in terms of numbers, percentage, rate and ratio.
2. **Impact indicators:** Can be used to monitor and measure progress of vendors to achieve the expected results/tender requirements as these indicators can measure the impact on addressing the specific procurement need/challenge. For example, indicators that measure increased energy efficiency or improved sustainability in an energy/environmental procurement or reduction of contamination in a healthcare procurement.

The results and indicators should be checked on *measurable*, *independently verifiable*, *realistic* and *achievable* data. Identifying the means of verification should take place in a coordinated manner when planning projects. Keep in mind that clear means of verification facilitate the establishment of monitoring and ex-post impact assessment systems and contributes significantly to ensuring evaluation.

9. ENSURE A MULTIDISCIPLINARY AND STRONGLY COMMITTED TEAM

Having a multidisciplinary team in your organisation and a strong senior management commitment is vital to implement an Innovation Procurement project. A procurement team is responsible for acquisition process of an organisation. The team is involved in the identification of needs, the establishment of budgets and the decision-making process. The procurement team can include representatives from different departments within the organisation.

Procurement teams help streamline the purchasing process by working together to find and describe the needs and procurement challenges. A well-functioning procurement team can save your organisation time and money. One of the main responsibilities of a procurement team is establishing budgets and working on a business case. This allows them to ensure that the best value for money solutions is purchased to achieve the organisation's goals and objectives.

To make effective purchasing decisions, a procurement team must have accurate information about the market conditions at hand. They need access to relevant data so they can make informed decisions. Generating trust with suppliers is also important for a successful procurement team as they may need to be able to share confidential information with these organisations.

Procurement teams play a vital role in ensuring that the organisation's business case is realised. They are actively involved in the preparation of the procurement, the tender process, the contracting and the performance monitoring to ensure quality and affordability. In addition, procurement teams can help reduce costs by applying contract performance clauses such as value engineering.

10. TAKE INTO ACCOUNT THAT YOUR PROJECT WILL TAKE TIME AND EFFORT

The planning phase of public procurement includes different steps/tasks, from the needs assessment to the state-of-the-art analysis and the market consultation, as well as the definition of functional and technical specifications, cost and pricing questions and the choice of procurement procedures.

The description of roles and responsibilities to carry out these tasks is necessary to ensure the optimal execution of the plans. The procurement team should assess the required time and effort needed from the team to achieve the project's objectives. The organisation should define in advance the capacity and resources needed to implement an Innovation Procurement project by establishing a timeline and clear milestones, as well as the person hours needed to complete the different tasks.

CLOSING REMARKS

The fast evolution of the society and the generation of new problems and needs in the health sector that cannot be addressed with the solutions available in the market leaves clear space for innovation. Although, traditionally, public buyers have been reluctant to purchase innovation due to the lack of experience and the potential risks involved, over time, they are becoming aware of the important benefits that this approach can bring to their organisation.

To successfully implement an Innovation Procurement the preparatory actions are particularly relevant and public buyers should spend time and resources to do so. The decision-making process should start within the organisation when identifying and prioritising the needs, researching the market and analysing the potential costs and benefits of the project. Then, the interaction with the market is essential to receive feedback and gain knowledge. Based on this interaction, the public buyer will be able to design the procurement strategy and set up an adequate mechanism to monitor contract execution. In any case, these steps require a strong commitment at the managerial level, a multidisciplinary team dedicated to the project and the allocation of time and effort.

REFERENCES

1. European Assistance For Innovation Procurement (EAFIP). www.eafip.eu
2. European Assistance for Innovation Procurement, "Eafip Toolkit." Available at: https://eafip.eu/toolkit/ (accessed: 2 August 2023).

FURTHER READING

European Commission, *Communication on Pre-commercial Procurement: Driving innovation to ensure sustainable high quality public services in Europe*. Brussels, 14.12.2007, COM (2007) 799 final. https://eur-lex.europa.eu/legal-content/EN/TXT/?uri=CELEX%3A52007DC0799R-Lex - 52007DC0799 - EN - EUR-Lex

European Commission, *Guidance on Innovation Procurement*. Brussels, 18.6.2021, C (2021) 4320 final.https://eur-lex.europa.eu/legal-content/EN/TXT/PDF/?uri=oj:JOC_2021_267_R_0001

European Commission, "Innovation Procurement." Available at: https://single-market-economy.ec.europa.eu/single-market/public-procurement/strategic-procurement/innovation-procurement_en (accessed: 10 August 2023).

European Commission, "Pre-Commercial Procurement." Available at: https://digital-strategy.ec.europa.eu/en/policies/pre-commercial-procurement (accessed: 10 August 2023).

5

A Guide to a Well-Founded Market Analysis for a Successful Open Market Consultation

Nazan Aynur and Karsten. W. Lemke

INTRODUCTION

Public clients such as clinics or care facilities often face the problem in their procurement projects that they do not know the market of potential bidders and their service portfolio exactly. There are recognised needs for which solutions are not (yet) offered on the market. In these cases, it is not only permissible but also advisable to conduct a market survey or analysis before initiating a procurement procedure.

In this chapter, we provide a condensed guide for newcomers in the field of public Innovation Procurement to carry out a well-founded market analysis with the aim of using the results of the analysis for a subsequent Open Market Consultation (OMC). Without this sound analysis, a subsequent consultation of relevant market participants for products, processes, solutions or even suggestions for improvement or ideas for the planning of research or development projects in the subject area of interest would not be successful or only insufficiently successful.

Before the contracting authority can start an award procedure, preparatory measures must be taken. Above all it is crucial to finalise the decision-making process for the specific service the client truly desires. The client must carry out a needs analysis and have answered the question: "What service do I actually want or need?"

This is an internal process in which the solution providers are not normally involved. In many cases, the client knows exactly what service they need. For example, if they want to outsource cleaning services, they know which buildings are to be cleaned, in which way and at what intervals. However, there are also many procurement projects in which the client faces problems precisely analysing these requirements. They may know what problem they want to solve with a particular procurement, but they do not know what solutions the market and potential bidders can offer them.

The market and the solutions available on the market, such as in the Information Technology (IT) sector, often develop so quickly that clients do not even know which options and solutions are available and which are still under development or close to market maturity. The same problem arises when the client wants to procure a service that does not yet exist on the market and must be produced for them.

In such cases, the client is unable to draw up a performance specification due to a lack of expertise. Nor can it define adequate eligibility and award criteria. Ultimately, it cannot estimate the value of the contract because it cannot know at what price and at what cost it will be able to meet its needs on the market. In each of these scenarios, conducting a procurement-related market analysis before initiating the award procedure is not only correct but also crucially important.

CONTENT DEVELOPMENT AND LEARNINGS

Step 1: Identification of Needs

The starting point of a well-founded market analysis is the identification of an "unmet need" in a specific subject area. This identified need is then broken down into one or more specific sample or use cases. In this chapter, we focus on a hospital wastewater (HWW) use case and take a closer look at the specific requirements and challenges of this aspect of sustainability. The requirements for an approach to needs identification have been described in chapter 3.

Step 2: Breaking Down into Use Cases

In the next step, it is important to break down the needs defined in the previous process into sample or use cases that are as concrete as possible. The use cases determined in this way must then be verified by the stakeholders and procurers. Only when this has been done can the actual market exploration or analysis take place.

EXAMPLE: ON-SITE TREATMENT OF HOSPITAL WASTEWATER

Context

Hospital wastewater (HWW) poses a significant environmental and health risk due to the presence of medicines, pharmaceuticals, pathogens and other hazardous substances. Traditional wastewater treatment methods employed by hospitals are often inadequate in effectively removing these contaminants.

Scope of the problem

Hospitals discharge considerable amounts of chemicals and microbial agents in their wastewaters. Problem chemicals present in hospital wastewater belong to different groups, such as antibiotics, X-ray contrast agents, disinfectants and pharmaceuticals. Many of these chemical compounds resist normal wastewater treatment.

Use case

On-site system, capable of effectively removing toxic substances, infectious compounds, pharmaceutical residues and pathogens from hospital wastewater.

Keywords

- Hospital wastewater treatment
- Innovative wastewater treatment technology
- Pharmaceutical wastewater treatment
- Pathogen removal in wastewater
- Advanced disinfection systems
- Contaminant removal in hospital wastewater
- Hospital wastewater pre-treatment
- Greenhouse gas reduction in wastewater treatment
- Regulated wastewater discharge systems
- Chemical-free wastewater treatment
- Microbial inactivation in hospital wastewater
- Residue removal in hospital wastewater

Situation

As is now: Due to the presence of medicines, pharmaceuticals, pathogens and other hazardous substances in HWW there is an environmental and health risks posed on the environment and the public.
Desirable situation: With an improved wastewater treatment system, the discharge from hospitals would have a reduced environmental impact through the discharging toxic substances, infectious compounds, pharmaceutical residues and pathogens into the environment or municipal water and minimise the risks on public health by ensuring the removal of disease-causing agents from hospital wastewater (the risk of waterborne transmission would be reduced and potential outbreaks or contamination of drinking water sources.)

Six steps to achieve "desirable state":

- Identify all the sources of HWW discharges within your hospital.
- Determine the types of healthcare pollutants present at each of the identified disposal channels.
- Familiarise yourself with the national and EU regulations and guidelines governing the discharge of HWW.
- Determine how the innovative solution can be integrated into your existing wastewater management system.
- Train relevant staff members on the operation, maintenance, and monitoring procedures of the new wastewater treatment system.
- Regular sampling and analysis of treated wastewater and regular assessing the performance of the wastewater treatment system and identify opportunities for optimisation and improvement to ensure integrated system meet the expected outcomes.

Step 3: Market Analysis

The market analysis consists of several coordinated sub-steps.

Desk Research

Carrying out comprehensive research using existing scientific databases (e.g. ebscohost.com, sciencedirect.com etc.), specialised literature and online resources. The aim is to collect and structure existing knowledge and information on the product/process for which the procurement requirement exists. It is best to ask yourself a few questions relating to the objectives and requirements of the planned procurement that will accompany the desk research process (see checklist below).

CHECKLIST

- What is the technical status of the solutions available on the market?
- What is the target (desired) status of the requested solution?
- Which functional requirements should be fulfilled?
- Is external technology and/or market knowledge necessary to precisely define the requirements?
- Are the requirements clearly and unambiguously formulated, or do they correspond to the language of the market?
- Which market players are potential suppliers?
- What potential solutions are available on the market?

The critical examination of existing and the formulation of new solution requirements is an important part of Innovation Procurement. These should be defined functionally and not target a specific technical solution, as the market should be given the opportunity to propose different solutions for the subsequent procurement process.

Discussions with Experts

Direct dialogue with experts from a specific subject area also makes it possible to gain insights into the state of the art in research and technology and to identify current market developments. These discussions help to close potential gaps in existing knowledge. It is advisable to diversify the group of experts interviewed in relation to their organisation or institution. The experts interviewed may come from:

- Universities/colleges.
- Other research institutions.
- Associations (e.g. in the case of the "hospital wastewater" use case, water supply and wastewater disposal associations or wastewater treatment plant associations).
- Government agencies (for water supply/water disposal/sewage treatment plants).
- Companies that offer solutions.

Attendance at Trade Fairs, Symposia and Themed Events

In addition to the discussions with experts described above, participation in trade fairs offers the opportunity to gain an overview of current trends, innovations and products on the market. Initial contacts with potential suppliers can also be made here.

Analysing the Products and Processes Available on the Market

A detailed analysis of what is available on the market, be it products, processes, services or business models, is crucial. This enables the identification of existing solutions and potential gaps in the market.

Analysing Patents and Standards: State-of-the-Art

A comprehensive prior search is carried out by analysing the current patent situation and searching for existing standards, both national and international, in the relevant subject area. This helps to understand the technological development and the legal framework.

With the help of patent analyses using patent databases such as DEPATISnet [1] in Germany or by consulting with patent experts, it is possible to determine which countries or regions have been very active in developing and patenting solutions. If, for example, a region shows hardly any relevant patent activities, this can be an indicator for innovation to be developed. For the individual steps of the market analysis, it is helpful to ask yourself a few questions, which we have summarised in the following checklist.

CHECKLIST

- Are there new, innovative (technical) solutions, processes or contractual design options for the specific requirements of procurement?
- What stage of development have these innovations reached?
- Are there potential solutions that will reach market maturity in the short to medium term, that is, within the next twelve months?
- Have promising providers been identified who have extensive technological experience or can provide a detailed (technical) description of a potential solution?
- Are there indications of possible improvements (costs, benefits) of these innovative solutions compared to conventional products (e.g. financial savings, energy efficiency, safety, social aspects, etc.)?
- Is there information on positive environmental impacts (e.g. less pollution, noise, disposal, etc.)?
- Which measurement parameters, norms, calculations, test procedures and standards should be considered and applied in the tender documents to inform the comparability of tenders?
- How can the life cycle costs (LCC) be calculated?
- Have the functional requirements been further specified?
- Has the market information been critically scrutinised and verified by independent parties (universities, research institutes, etc.)?

In addition to the five sub-steps described above, there are other ways of broadening the engagement for the market analysis in focus. These include:

Obtaining Written Offers

Suppliers may be requested to submit non-binding offers containing the following information:

- Technical details and functionalities.
- Information on possible savings potential of the technical solution (energy, maintenance, acquisition costs, etc.).
- Development stage and market readiness of the solution or product.

- Cost estimate or indication.
- Potential risks.
- Conformity with applied standards.

The information obtained must not be used to exclude suppliers from the actual tender. In addition, confidentiality agreements are often required between the parties to protect critical data from being passed on.

Open Seminars and Workshops

Open dialogue with potential suppliers can clarify important issues. As this dialogue is public, technical and confidential details and pricing information are usually kept in confidence.

Closed Discussions

This very direct form of communication is conducted with potential suppliers individually and confidentially. It is very effective but requires urgent adherence to basic principles such as transparency, non-discrimination and equal treatment of suppliers. Consequently, the process and results of such meetings should be documented, and the results should not lead to the exclusion or favouring of individual suppliers.

Regardless of whether for open seminars, workshops or closed discussions, framework criteria should be observed:

a. **Selection of participants in the consultation process:** In order not to disadvantage any company, all interested providers/suppliers should be invited to participate in the consultation. It is important that the participants have expertise in evaluating technical details and can assess the effects and risks for the organisation. Representatives from research institutes and universities can also be invited to the consultations. They bring scientific aspects to the discussion and provide valuable information on the state of development and degree of innovation of the technologies.
b. **Publication of the consultation results:** In the interests of transparency and equal treatment, the relevant results of the consultation rounds should be published without breaching the confidentiality of detailed information. Publication marks the end of this process step.

Step 4: Summarising the results

The final step before conducting an Open Market Consultation is to review and collate the researched facts and results from the various parts of the market analysis. This enables the creation of a comprehensive picture of existing offers, innovative solutions, challenges and potential gaps in the market. The OMC can then be prepared with the help of a "market report".

Step 5: Open Market Consultation

The summarised results serve as the starting point and basis for the Open Market Consultation. This phase enables a wide range of stakeholders to contribute their perspectives, ideas and concerns. The OMC is an important step to further validate the market and confirm the need for innovative solutions.

CLOSING REMARKS

The guidance for a well-founded market analysis for a successful Open Market Consultation is a decisive contribution to the development of sustainable solutions. A systematic approach, starting with the identification of needs through to open consultation, creates a solid foundation for the development of innovative products and services. This chapter provides valuable guidance for all stakeholders who want to actively participate in shaping sustainable markets.

REFERENCE

1. Datenbank zu Patentveröffentlichungen aus aller Welt: https://depatisnet.dpma.de/

6

Why Open Market Consultation (OMC) Is Crucial to Innovation Procurement

Ana Lucia Jaramillo Villacís, Beatriz Gómez Fariñas and Azra Atalan

INTRODUCTION

As previously noted, public procurement represents around 14% of GDP in the EU, thus it has the potential to drive innovation and improve the quality and efficiency of public services. Before launching a procurement procedure, public procurers may conduct market consultations for preparing the procurement and informing economic operators of their procurement plans and requirements. Understanding what the market can offer is fundamental to knowing how to steer an Innovation Procurement project.

Innovation Procurement is a tool public buyers can use to acquire the development or deployment of pioneering innovative solutions to address specific mid-to-long-term public sector needs. This approach fosters innovation from the demand side and helps shape markets as well as create new ones, thus creating opportunities for small and medium enterprises (SMEs).

In this chapter, we explore the importance, methodology and best practices of an Open Market Consultation (OMC) in the preparatory phase of any Innovation Procurement project. The dialogue with the market is essential to inform economic operators in advance about the procurement plans and cross-check the findings on the State-Of-the Art (SOTA) analysis. The feedback from the market is useful to understand the capability of technology providers to solve the challenges identified and the feasibility of the Innovation Procurement envisaged. Interaction with the market can help clarify questions and identify blind spots of information. It also creates a sense of trust because of the transparency and openness in the presentation of the needs and plans from the public buyers who wish to consider the input from the market operators. To illustrate this, we present some example cases from the P4H project.

Innovation Procurement includes:

- The development of innovative solutions through the procurement of Research and Development (R&D) services. This is possible by conducting Pre-Commercial Procurement (PCP).
- The procurement of innovative solutions that are not yet available or do not exist on the market; or the procurement of innovative solutions that do exist but are not yet widely available on the market. In this case, the public buyer acts as a launching customer through Public Procurement of Innovative Solutions (PPI).
- A preparatory stage before launching a tender, which is essential to ensure the feasibility of the contract, the full satisfaction of the public buyer's needs and efficient spending of the public funds. In this context, the interaction with the market is a step without which public buyers face the risk of launching a tender, lacking sufficient knowledge of the market and failing to achieve the objectives of the Innovation Procurement project. Therefore, it is useful to strengthen the capabilities of public procurers in conducting legally sound market consultations that provide practical insights for future procurement.

The interaction with the market is an important step in the design and preparation of the contract and for the success of your Innovation Procurement project. Think, for example, about your own experience if you need to buy a new car for your family. You investigate the alternatives available on the market, perhaps you visit some showrooms to ask for information and read reviews and compare the features of the different types of cars that could fit the needs of your family. Imagine then how important it is to have insights from the market when you are planning to embark on a challenging project to obtain innovative solutions for the public sector. Of course, you need knowledge of what the market can offer. You really need to find out if there are solutions already available and commercialised or if it is feasible to develop what you need to solve a problem within the time and budget of your initial plan.

Therefore, you should pay special attention to how you communicate and interact with the market using a legally sound methodology, the right tools, and allocating the time and efforts required to conduct an OMC with EU-wide coverage. In this chapter, you will get a clear picture of the objectives of an OMC, the legal basis from a European perspective, how to announce an OMC and how to conduct it using specific tools, including a Request for Information (RFI) questionnaire.

WHAT IS AN OPEN MARKET CONSULTATION (OMC)?

An OMC is a procedure open to all interested parties who can provide valuable information about the market capabilities and readiness to participate in an Innovation Procurement project. Once you have a well-defined need that you intend to satisfy through Innovation Procurement, the next step is to explore whether this approach is suitable and under which conditions by exploring what the market can deliver and/or has in the R&D pipeline, by engaging with technology vendors and conducting a cost-benefit analysis with the feedback received. If this assessment shows that there are no solutions available in the market to fully meet your needs and the project is economically feasible, then it is possible to conduct an Innovation Procurement process.

The European Public Procurement Directives of 2014 regulate the preliminary market consultations in the sense that public procurers may conduct market consultations before the procurement in compliance with the principles of transparency, equal treatment and non-discrimination, without distorting competition.

In general, the objectives of the OMC are to:

- Validate the findings of the market and SoTA analysis as well as the viability of the set of technical and financial provisions.
- Raise awareness of the industry and relevant stakeholders regarding the upcoming Innovation Procurement project.
- Collect insights from the industry and relevant stakeholders (including end users) to fine tune the tender specifications.

The OMC is performed under the law of the contracting authority (or the lead procurer in a joint procurement). The contracting authority can set clear rules and objectives of the OMC. For example, it can state expressly in an OMC document that it is not legally bound in any way by the outcome of the OMC and that starting an OMC does not mean that the contracting authority will start a tendering or purchasing procedure. There is a clear separation between the OMC and the tendering procedure.

The target groups for an OMC are usually technology providers and end users. All interested parties are invited to take part in an OMC on a voluntary and non-binding basis, generally at the own expense and risk of market operators. In an OMC, it can be announced clearly that market operators cannot charge any costs for participation in the OMC or for (re-) use of the information in the context of a future procurement procedure.

The OMC is not part of any pre-qualification or selection process. No advantage or disadvantage is given to any technology provider or group of technology providers to the detriment of others during the OMC and the subsequent competitive procedure for the award of contracts. Participation in an OMC is not a condition for submitting a tender in the subsequent procurement, does not lead to any rights or privileges for the participants, and the input provided in an OMC is not used to evaluate future proposals. For the widest reach it is recommended that where possible the information provided during the OMC and other background information are provided in English.

EXTRACT FROM AN OMC DOCUMENT IN PROCURE4HEALTH

Through this OMC, the Public Buyers Group (PBG) of Procure4Health (identified in section 2), with *Reseau Des Acheteurs Hospitaliers IDF* (RESAH) as lead procurer, aims to challenge the market to develop innovative solutions to effectively remove toxic substances, infectious compounds, pharmaceutical residues, and pathogens from hospital wastewater (HWW) on the hospital's premises.

Nowadays, hospitals discharge considerable amounts of chemicals and microbial agents in their wastewater, such as antibiotics, X-ray contrast agents, disinfectants, and pharmaceuticals. Many of these chemical compounds resist normal wastewater treatment. The presence of those substances in HWW poses an environmental and health risk (e.g. the risk of waterborne transmission and potential outbreaks or contamination of drinking water sources).

In this context, the purpose of the OMC is to inform technology providers and other relevant stakeholders about the needs of the PBG and to gather their input about the Procure4Health challenge for developing a solution to sanitise HWW on-site with the following required functionalities:

- Channelling the HWW into a centralised treatment facility.
- Separating/treating highly soluble reagents like sodium azide or other hazardous chemicals.
- Removing large solid debris and coarse materials from the wastewater.
- Working stably despite high concentrations of disinfection agents.
- Treating persistent organic pollutants.
- Meeting the required wastewater discharge standards by disinfecting HWW.
- Reducing nutrient concentrations (like nitrogen and phosphorus).
- Filtering and separating HWW through advanced treatment technologies.
- Handling properly any sludge that might form.
- Including monitoring devices and sensors to measure important parameters like pH, temperature, dissolved oxygen and pollutant concentrations.
- Odour control.
- If possible, depending on local regulations and requirements, reusing the treated HWW for non-potable applications within the hospital, such as irrigation, toilet flushing or cooling tower makeup water.

Another objective of the OMC is to understand the technology providers' capabilities to satisfy the public buyers' needs and to obtain their input on the viability of the procurement plans and conditions as described in this document and annexes [1].

HOW TO ANNOUNCE AN OMC?

One of the best practices to ensure the principles of transparency, equal treatment and non-discrimination, and to achieve EU-wide outreach, is to publish a PIN in the European portal Tenders Electronics Daily (TED). However, once the PIN has been published, additional outreach activities through relevant networks are desirable to enhance the dissemination of the OMC and the participation of relevant stakeholders. In addition to the publication of the PIN, another best practice is to make available an OMC document, providing information about the project and setting the rules of the OMC.

The findings of the market consultation are published in the form of an OMC Report to ensure that the parties who did not participate in the market consultation are also informed about the procedure and the results obtained. It could be that national legislation establishes additional reporting requirements, so it is important to verify which information you must make available based on your legislation. From the EU perspective, there is not a specific format nor requirements concerning what the report should contain. Therefore, it can be a report with anonymised data and a set of conclusions.

WHAT KIND OF ACTIVITIES DO YOU CONDUCT IN AN OMC?

The OMC may take the form of an on-site and/or online event, combined with a Request for Information (RFI) questionnaire using free tools like EU Survey.

The event or webinar can be recorded and made available on a website. For example, the video recordings from this OMC are available on the website of Procure4Health [1]. After processing and analysing the answers to the questionnaire, the results are disseminated to the widest possible audience through an OMC report.

UNDERSTANDING WHAT THE MARKET CAN OFFER

Conducting an EU-wide market consultation announced in the TED through a PIN can provide the basis for starting a procurement. The market consultation is important in several ways:

- It enables you to cross-check the market analysis previously performed and helps validate the innovation potential of the need.

- It provides feedback on how to raise interest from the market to answer the upcoming call for tender, the type of players on the market and what they can offer.
- It makes potentially interested bidders aware of the public procurers' needs.
- It allows cross-checking the feasibility and market acceptance of the envisaged contract set-up (key contractual conditions, budget, timeframe, etc.).

To achieve these objectives, there are some aspects that you need to consider:

- Communicate the identified needs openly and clearly to all potentially interested bidders (including the costs of the existing solution and the results of the market analysis).
- Mention your desire for an innovative outcome in the announcement of the market consultation.
- Give the suppliers sufficient time to ask questions and provide their views on the progress of ongoing product development and the feasibility of the proposed procurement approach.
- Identify the right market segments and disseminate the market consultation effectively, well in advance to ensure broad participation.
- Guarantee the security of confidential information, trade secrets and intellectual property.

CLOSING REMARKS

To implement an Innovation Procurement successfully, the preparatory actions are particularly important, and public buyers should spend time and resources to complete these. The decision-making process should start within the organisation when identifying and prioritising the needs, researching the market and analysing the potential costs and benefits of the project. Interaction with the market is essential to receive feedback and gain knowledge for future procurement. Based upon this interaction, the public buyer will be able to design the procurement strategy and set up adequate mechanisms to monitor the contract execution.

A market consultation should comply with the principles of transparency, equal treatment and non-discrimination to ensure that there is no distortion of competition in the future tender. There are different activities which can be covered by the OMC, for example on-site and/or online events where the public buyers engage in a dialogue with technology providers to obtain feedback concerning their capabilities and readiness to respond to the challenges and functional requirements described in use cases, as well as to receive input on the feasibility of the envisaged procurement plans, including the conditions regarding the management of intellectual property rights, the budget and timeline foreseen.

The publication of an OMC document and the respective OMC report summarising the findings and conclusions can provide a good basis to understand the objectives, the rules and the results of the activities conducted, for any interested party who may participate in the future Innovation Procurement process, even if it did not participate in the OMC. The

Table 6.1 Example of the timetable of an OMC from the first challenge of the Procure4Health project

Date	Event
5 January	Publication of the general Prior Information Notice (PIN) on TED: https://ted.europa.eu/en/notice/-/detail/6662-2024
March	Publication of the PIN on TED (specific for this challenge): https://ted.europa.eu/en/notice/-/detail/185487-2024
4 March	Publication of the OMC documents on the project's website: https://procure4health.eu/omc-on-site-treatment-of-hospital-wastewater/ Publication of the EU Survey questionnaire: https://ec.europa.eu/eusurvey/runner/Procure4Health-water-treatment
3 April	OMC Event in English (online) (10:00–11:30 CET). Webinar recording: https://youtu.be/5kGguQdv6c8?feature=shared
18 April	Deadline for the submission of questions via the OMC questionnaire (17:00 CET).
6 May	Publication of the OMC findings, including all questions and answers to the OMC questionnaire: https://procure4health.eu/wp-content/uploads/2024/05/Procure4Health_OMC-Report_HWW_final.pdf
8 May	Closure of the OMC.

OMC is crucial to an Innovation Procurement project because it helps public buyers/contracting authorities make informed decisions for the future procurement process.

REFERENCE

1. https://procure4health.eu/omc-on-site-treatment-of-hospital-wastewater/

FURTHER READING

Articles 40 and 41 of Directive 2014/24/EU of the European Parliament and of the Council of 26 February 2014 on public procurement and repealing Directive 2004/18/EC. https://eur-lex.europa.eu/eli/dir/2014/24/oj/eng.

European Commission, *Communication on Pre-commercial Procurement: Driving Innovation to Ensure Sustainable High Quality Public Services in Europe*. Brussels, 14.12.2007, COM (2007) 799 final. https://eur-lex.europa.eu/legal-content/EN/TXT/?uri=CELEX:52007DC0799.

European Commission, *Guidance on Innovation Procurement*. Brussels, 18.6.2021, C (2021) 4320 final. https://op.europa.eu/s/z6W3.

European Commission, "Innovation Procurement." Available at: https://single-market-economy.ec.europa.eu/single-market/public-procurement/strategic-procurement/innovation-procurement_en (accessed: 10 August 2023).

European Commission, "Pre-Commercial Procurement." Available at: https://digital-strategy.ec.europa.eu/en/policies/pre-commercial-procurement (accessed: 10 August 2023).

European portal Tenders Electronics Daily (TED). https://ted.europa.eu/en/.

Open Market Consultations in the context of Procure4Health. https://procure4health.eu/open-market-consultation/.

7

Key Aspects to Consider When Evaluating the Offers in Your Pre-Commercial Procurement (PCP) Tender

Klaus Piesche, Sonja Müller and Lutz Kubitschke

INTRODUCTION

There are two big differences between a standard tender and a Pre-Commercial Procurement (PCP) tender: in PCPs you procure Research and Development (R&D) rather than a product that already is available on the market, and as a PCP involves multiple phases, the evaluation may need to be adapted as the project progresses. The process for creating a PCP tender have been considered in depth in earlier chapters. Here, we focus on the evaluation phase of the tender.

There are five key factors to be assessed during a PCP tender evaluation:

1. **Relevance to the objectives:** Evaluate how well the tender addresses the specific goals and challenges outlined in your PCP call. The applicant should demonstrate a clear understanding of the problem and offer solutions that are directly aligned with your PCP's needs.
2. **Technical feasibility and quality:** Assess the technical soundness of the proposed solution. This includes the feasibility of the approach, the robustness of the methodology, and the likelihood of achieving the desired outcomes within the project timeline.
3. **Innovation and quality:** Determine the level of innovation presented in the tender. The tenderer should offer novel ideas and/or approaches that go beyond the current state of the art, providing added value and potential breakthroughs in the field.
4. **Capability and expertise:** Examine the qualifications, experience and competencies of the team behind the tender.
5. **Value for money:** Consider the cost-effectiveness of the proposal. Evaluate whether the proposed budget is reasonable and provides good value in relation to the benefits and outcomes expected.

In addition to these five assessment factors, we have learnt from experience that there are eight aspects that require attention for successful evaluation.

Aspect 1: Keep the Evaluation in Mind When Writing Tender Documents

When crafting your tender documents, it's essential to consider the evaluation process from the outset. That usually helps you to set requirements that are not only clear and reasonably concise but also in some way measurable, making life easier for both evaluators and potential suppliers.

To simplify, imagine there are three types of requirements, sorted by how easy they are to evaluate:

- **Type 1** (easiest to evaluate): Binary, Yes/No requirements. Straightforward and little-to-no room for subjective interpretation. Example: *"The solution must be compatible with devices running on Android and iOS operating systems."*
- **Type 2** (moderately easy to evaluate): Quantitative or measurable requirements. Require more detail but can still be verified objectively by comparing with predefined criteria. Example: *"The solution must support at least x concurrent users without performance degradation, as measured by industry-standard load testing tools."*
- **Type 3** (hardest to evaluate): Qualitative or subjective requirements. Assessments based on the quality, user experience, or innovative aspects; often relying on the evaluator's judgment. Example: *"The solution must provide an intuitive user interface that enhances user experience and allows for seamless navigation across all features."*

As your tender should allow the suppliers sufficient leeway to be innovative, shifting the focus onto WHAT is expected rather than HOW to achieve it: you will not only have to deal extensively with Type 3 requirements but also formulate your Type 1 and Type 2 requirements in such a way that they do not overly limit the suppliers.

On a positive note, in PCPs where you are procuring R&D, Type three requirements usually tend to get easier to evaluate in later phases, when prototypes become available and initial feasibility and prototype tests have taken place: provided your evaluation committee members are aware of these developments and have a reasonable understanding of the outcomes. For more on the evaluation committee, please see Aspect 3.

Aspect 2: Decide on the Granularity and Weighting of Your Evaluation Criteria

Eventually, you will have to translate your requirements into a set of clear evaluation criteria to include in the tender documents. Again, there will be choices to make regarding the granularity of your evaluation criteria: does every single requirement get assigned a weight or does it make more sense to group requirements and assign weights per group?

Consider the complexity of your requirements and the objectives of your evaluation process to decide which method, or combination of methods, will provide the most effective and fair assessment of the tenders. Often, a blended approach works best.

Assign weights to individual requirements when:

- Your PCP has critical requirements that must be met with precision.
- You need to differentiate between the importance of specific features.
- A detailed evaluation is necessary for compliance reasons.

Group requirements and assign single weights when:

- Your PCP encompasses many requirements that can be (logically) categorised.
- You aim for a more holistic evaluation of your proposals.
- Efficiency and simplicity are priorities for the evaluation process.

If you opt to keep the same set of evaluation criteria for all three phases (as we have in most of our PCPs), consider keeping the weights for these criteria flexible throughout the phases to align with phase-specific goals as the PCP progresses. For example, in Phase 1 you may want to place the highest weight on innovativeness and understanding of the problem you want to tackle with your PCP, whereas you would shift the weights towards implementation in Phase 3. Alternatively, it's perfectly acceptable to have different evaluation criteria in each phase as well. The key is to communicate clearly the criteria for each phase to your potential suppliers.

Aspect 3: Assemble an Evaluation Committee with Relevant Expertise in Due Time before the Evaluation Starts, to avoid Conflicts of Interest

Internal Evaluation Committee versus External Evaluation Committee

Why choose an internal evaluation committee? Internal evaluation committee members might be more familiar with the procurement objectives and the context within which the PCP operates. They can provide a sort of continuity throughout the procurement process, especially if they have been involved in earlier stages, for example, in drafting the tender documents or being part of the requirements engineering group. Costs are lower since internal staff are already employed. However, internal staff usually have other duties, which may limit their capacity to dedicate sufficient time to the evaluation.

> *An intermediate model is an internal evaluation committee with an added expert board or technical panel supporting the evaluation committee.*

Technical panels can add significant value to the evaluation process by leveraging their specialised knowledge, especially for cutting-edge technologies. When assessing the technological offerings in detail, they can help to distinguish effectively between substantive information and less relevant or overly complex technical descriptions. This especially holds true for emerging technologies such as AI. While AI has the potential to deliver transformative solutions, their inclusion in proposals often lacks the necessary substantiation to demonstrate practical applicability or alignment with project objectives. It is therefore crucial to evaluate their relevance critically, ensuring their use is driven by tangible value and feasibility.

Your tender has been published; your evaluation committee is all set and now the only thing left to do (this might be not entirely true) is to evaluate the numerous tenders you have received. There is one important thing to do before you start into the evaluation, regardless of the approach you choose: make sure that no member of your evaluation committee or any supplementary board has a conflict of interest: none whatsoever. In most cases potential conflicts become apparent only after the tenders have been opened. Discovering even a potential conflict too late in the process can seriously impact the timeline of your evaluations.

Identifying conflicts of interest is not always straightforward. For example, a member of your evaluation committee is a professor in the Faculty of Medicine, Department of Geriatrics, at a French University. If a tenderer includes another Professor from the same University and faculty as the project advisor, even if she works in a different department and building, this could be perceived as a potential conflict of interest. Although this situation might seem indirect, it is important to consider such connections to maintain the integrity of the evaluation process.

Aspect 4: Document Everything Thoroughly

Documenting everything thoroughly during the tender phase and evaluation is crucial for several reasons. While being compliant with regulations and having a defence against possible challenges is an obvious reason, documentation can also be useful as a means of preserving knowledge. Detailed records help to ensure continuity, particularly if team members change. In a PCP, where lessons learnt from previous phases and evaluations can help shape the call-off tender documents, documenting what worked (and what did not) will assist in making the tendering procedures smoother, more efficient, and less prone to issues. It can help to think of thorough documentation less as a bureaucratic burden and more of a survival tool: it will be your safety net, your evidence and your saving grace.

Aspect 5: Consistent Communication

One aspect of transparency is to communicate consistently. To start with, provide a clear explanation of the evaluation process in the tender documents. This should include comprehensive information on evaluation criteria and sub-criteria and their respective weightings, and what constitutes a satisfactory response.

For tender documents, communicate any changes to the tender process or timelines promptly to all participants. If you have the tender documents on your website, it can make sense to ask for an email address before allowing downloads. That way, you know whom to contact and inform about updates. In one PCP we asked interested downloaders either to provide their real email address or, if they did not want any more information, simply to enter *dontbotherme@project.name*. Twenty per cent of people did this, and we did send them unsolicited emails.

If you make changes to your tender documents, let users know about the changes in a change log. This can be a simple .txt file added to your tender documents' library. A change log also makes it easier for you to track all changes, and you can include the changes directly on your website.

Provide clear contact information for queries throughout the process, from the initial tender up until Phase three. In our experience clarification Meetings with question-and-answer sessions have been valuable, and the outcomes were disseminated to all interested parties either via the website (for Phase one) or in the collaborative workspace of suppliers and procurers. Along the same lines, allow a period for tenderers to submit questions and share response with all participants.

Keep records of all communications between tenderers (and later suppliers) and procurers and make all information equally available to all tenderers/suppliers to prevent misinformation. Ideally, there should be only one single point of contact to make life easier for everyone.

Aspect 6: Scoring Is Only Half the Work

After each round of evaluation, it is good practice to offer evaluation summaries explaining to unsuccessful tenderers why their proposals were not selected. If you have many proposals, this can entail a significant amount of work. Therefore, prepare your evaluation committee not only to assign scores but also to provide one or two sentences explaining what led them to these scores. You can later compile this information for the outcome letters.

The same applies to successful tenderers: by providing meaningful insights into the strengths and weaknesses of their proposals, you help them to improve their offers for the next phases. Instead of a vague comment like *"data collection approach is not good"* a more meaningful comment would be, for example: *"the approach of using ducks with cameras to collect patient data is not effective, as patients might be allergic to poultry and the download would be too heavy for a commercially available European duck."*

Aspect 7: Quality and Innovation in a Proposal *or* Be Aware of Too Much Innovation *or* Avoid the Pitfalls of Overcomplexity and Impracticality

Innovation should always address directly the challenges outlined in the tender documents and not overcomplicate the solution. Innovation should be a means to an end, not an end in itself. The reasons for this are many: technologies that are not yet validated and might be difficult to validate within the PCP; unforeseen technical hurdles; overengineering (adding multiple levels of complexity); user adoption issues; and infrastructure limitations (implementation!).

Aspect 8: Evaluating IPR Is Not Always an Easy Task

To simplify the evaluation process consider using an IPR framework template, including foreground Intellectual Property (IP) ownership, (the usual PCP rule is that the supplier retains the IP rights), usage rights for procurers, clearly defined terms for licensing rights (e.g. for internal use, testing, pilot deployments, sublicensing), and access to background IP rights.

Criteria might include the scope of licensing (are the usage rights for the procurers sufficient, fair, and clear?); commercialisation strategy (especially in the later phases: do they have a clear plan for exploiting the IPR beyond the PCP); risk mitigation and transparency (are third-party IP dependencies well documented and described to avoid potential access issues later); and reusability (do the proposed IPR terms allow for scaling or reuse across public procurers?).

Escrow agreements: While not directly tied to evaluation, you might consider including an escrow agreement in your tender documents. An escrow agreement allows a neutral third party to hold critical materials (e.g. prototypes, technical documentation, or source code) under predefined conditions. If the supplier fails to deliver or fulfil obligations (e.g. bankruptcy or abandonment), the procurer can access the escrowed materials for continuity without claiming ownership of the IPR. This approach aligns well with PCP guidelines by balancing supplier rights with risk mitigation for procurers.

Typically, IPR aspects can feel a bit shadowy in the beginning stages of PCP, largely because no product yet exists. In our experience, tools like an IPR framework template or escrow agreements can add a bit of clarity and confidence to the process.

GENERAL CONSIDERATION: YOU ARE NOT BUYING A TOASTER, YOU ARE BUYING THE FUTURE *OR*: "CHEAP TODAY" OFTEN MEANS "EXPENSIVE TOMORROW"

In our opinion "traditional" criteria such as "lowest phase price" are not the most suitable approach in a PCP, as they tend to create an evaluation process that risks failing to reward quality, sustainability, or long-term value. PCP is about investing in solutions that deliver the most value, not the lowest price. If you want to keep the future-you from screaming into a pillow, we recommend concentrating on Value-Based Procurement (VBP (see chapter 9) and cost-effectiveness over the solution's lifecycle. And as we are talking about *the future*: why not also evaluate the environmental sustainability (chapter 8)?

What Is There to Evaluate Regarding Cost-effectiveness?

- Total cost of ownership (TCO): Assess all costs, including R&D, deployment, maintenance, and operational costs.
- Performance *vs.* cost: Does the proposed solution improve efficiency, reduce waste, or streamline processes in a way that justifies its cost?
- Impact on resources: Will the proposed solution save time, labour or other resources for the procurer?
- Scalability costs: Can the proposed solution be implemented more widely or reused without significant additional investment?

Value-Based procurement: A brief mention of VBP, as this is considered in detail in chapter 9. VBP shifts the focus from *lowest cost* to *highest value*, prioritising outcomes that deliver long-term benefits for people and systems. In the healthcare sector that could mean:

- Patient outcomes: Will the proposed solution improve patient care, health outcomes or quality of life?
- Cost savings for healthcare systems: Does the proposed solution reduce hospital stays, improve diagnostics, or lower the need for interventions?

With respect to environmental sustainability, there are a handful of things to consider:

- Carbon footprint: Does the proposed solution reduce energy consumption or emissions?
- Resource efficiency: Does the proposed solution use materials efficiently (this could be difficult to evaluate) or minimise waste (e.g. recyclability or using modular components)?
- Lifecycle environmental impact: What are the environmental costs across the solution's design, production, use, and disposal phases?
- Does the proposed solution promote the reuse, repair, recycling principles of the Circular Economy?
- Do suppliers have credible sustainability policies or certifications?

CLOSING REMARKS

PCP processes can feel daunting, even for seasoned professionals. In this chapter, we aimed to break down the evaluation process into digestible, actionable steps, showcasing key aspects, such as aligning requirements with evaluation criteria, weighing innovation against practicality and maintain transparency throughout.

Whilst PCPs come with unique challenges, they also unlock opportunities to drive innovation in public procurement, particularly within healthcare. By learning from past experiences and tailoring approaches to the nuances of PCPs collectively we can enhance procurement strategies, yielding better outcomes for both procurers and end-users: patients whose lives these innovations ultimately are meant to improve.

8

A Practical Guide to Advancing Sustainable Procurement of Innovation

Ali Fakih

INTRODUCTION

The healthcare sector in Europe wields substantial purchasing power. This economic influence presents a unique opportunity to shape markets toward ethically produced, environmentally sustainable, and health-conscious products and services. While the integration of sustainability into procurement practices varies across European countries, many hospitals and health procurers are leveraging public funds to enhance community well-being, support healthier environments, and drive sustainable innovation.

Understanding the critical areas for success in sustainable Innovation Procurement is essential for transforming procurement from a transactional process into a strategic tool for positive change. By focusing on these areas, organisations can create a clear roadmap to address sustainability challenges while fostering innovation that delivers real impact.

This approach enables procurement to go beyond cost considerations, emphasising solutions that generate environmental, social, and economic value. It equips procurers with the ability to align with meeting sustainability goals, driving progress toward a more sustainable future through thoughtful, innovative decision-making.

> *"Strategic procurement is not just about purchasing goods and services; it's about leveraging every decision to create value, drive innovation, and build a sustainable future."*

By incorporating sustainability and innovation into procurement practices, organisations can align their operational goals with environmental, social, and economic priorities. For example, the European Commission estimates that sustainable public procurement could represent up to 14% of EU GDP, underlining its potential to shape both economic and environmental outcomes [1]. This approach highlights the key factors that drive success, offering practical insights into how organisations can create transformative solutions. It also stresses the importance of strategic alignment, leadership support, and collaboration to unlock procurement's potential as a driver of a more sustainable and equitable future. Moreover, companies with strong environmental, social and governance (ESG) credentials can reduce costs by 5–10%, as they focus on improving operational efficiency and reducing waste [2].

WHAT STRATEGIC PROCUREMENT DECISIONS LOOK LIKE

Strategic purchasing decisions are about moving beyond the traditional focus on price, quality and quantity. They involve making intentional choices that align with broader sustainability goals: environmental, social, and economic, while also fostering innovation. Here is what it could look like in practice:

Prioritising Sustainable Products and Services

Choosing eco-friendly, socially responsible and economically efficient products. Choose suppliers that offer products designed for reuse or repair; helping to reduce waste and support a circular economy.

Opting for Long-Term, Value-Driven Contracts

Instead of making decisions based solely on the lowest priced bid, strategic purchasing involves considering the long-term value. Look at the total cost of ownership, life cycle costing over the life of a product or service, rather than just the upfront price.

Leveraging Innovation to Drive Sustainability

Strategic purchasing encourages looking for innovative solutions that not only meet needs but also drive sustainability progress.

Partnering with Suppliers Who Share Sustainability Values

Selecting suppliers aligned with sustainability goals and fostering long-term partnerships. When selecting vendors, include sustainability criteria in the tender process.

This chapter focuses on a key strategic procurement decision: *leveraging innovation to drive sustainability.* This decision is critical for organisations looking to make a significant impact on sustainability, as it centres around fostering the development and adoption of innovative solutions that address environmental and social challenges.

THREE STEPS APPROACH: IDENTIFY – CHECK – DRIVE

The "identify–check the market–drive the market" cycle is a straightforward framework for advancing the sustainable procurement of innovation.

Step 1: Identify Sustainability Needs

The process of shifting innovation towards more sustainable solutions begins with identifying an "unmet need" in a specific area related to sustainability. This involves identifying areas where current practices fall short in reducing environmental impact, improving social outcomes, or enhancing economic efficiency. Once this need is recognised, it is further broken down into one or more specific use cases or examples that help clarify the solution required.

Identifying a sustainability need begins with recognising and clearly defining the underlying problem. For instance, in the case of polyvinyl chloride (PVC) usage in healthcare, the problem lies in its environmental and health impacts. The widespread reliance on PVC in medical devices and packaging has led to concerns about toxic chemical exposure during production, the leaching of harmful additives like phthalates, and the release of dangerous dioxins during incineration. These issues highlight an unmet need for safer, more sustainable materials.

By pinpointing this specific problem, we can identify the sustainability need: the development of alternative materials that maintain the functionality of PVC while eliminating its risks.

TIPS FOR SUCCESS

- Engage Healthcare Professionals and Departments: Collaborate with clinical staff, facility managers, procurement teams and other stakeholders to understand the environmental and social challenges specific to hospital operations and supply chains.
- Conduct Sustainability Audits: Perform assessments within the hospital to identify areas for improvement, such as energy efficiency in operating rooms, reduction of medical waste or ensuring ethical labour practices in the production of medical supplies.
- Involve Patients and Community Feedback: Gather input from patients and local communities to understand their perspectives on sustainability in healthcare services and identify areas where hospitals can make meaningful improvements.
- Define Sustainability Goals Clearly: Frame specific and measurable sustainability needs, such as reducing single-use plastics in medical devices or sourcing renewable energy for hospital operations, to inspire innovative solutions from suppliers and service providers.

Step 2: Check the Market

After identifying sustainability needs, the next step is to analyse the market landscape to uncover potential solutions. This involves assessing the availability of sustainable technologies, products, and suppliers that align with your goals. Within the healthcare context, this means exploring innovative materials, eco-friendly processes, and market leaders who demonstrate commitment to environmental and social responsibility. This step helps determine whether existing solutions can meet the identified needs or if there is a gap that requires driving innovation through collaboration with suppliers.

TIPS FOR SUCCESS

- Engage in Pre-Market Consultations: Organise meetings or workshops with potential suppliers to discuss your sustainability needs and understand what solutions they can offer. This dialogue can also inspire innovation tailored to your specific challenges.
- Collaborate Through Procurement Networks: Engage with networks like Global Green and Healthy Hospitals (GGHH) to collaborate with other procurers tackling similar sustainability challenges. These networks serve as platforms for sharing knowledge, learning from real-world experiences, and accessing case studies of solutions that have been tested and implemented.
- Analyse Market Readiness: Evaluate whether the market has mature solutions that meet your needs or if innovative approaches are still in development. This helps in deciding whether to pursue PCP or PPI strategies.
- Global Green and Healthy Hospitals (GGHH [3]: This is an international network of hospitals, healthcare facilities, health systems and health organisations dedicated to reducing their environmental footprint and promoting public and environmental health. The GGHH network has over 2,000 members in more than 80 countries who are using innovation, ingenuity, and investment to transform the health sector and foster a healthy, sustainable future.

Step 3: Drive the Market

Once sustainability needs are identified and the market has been assessed, the next step is to actively influence the market to deliver innovative, sustainable solutions. This involves working collaboratively with suppliers, setting clear and measurable sustainability criteria, and using procurement as a tool to push industries toward more environmentally and socially responsible practices.

By taking a leadership role, procurers can signal the demand for sustainable solutions and incentivise suppliers to innovate. In healthcare, this could mean requesting products that have a reduced carbon footprint; reduce use of unnecessary plastics, phase out toxic chemicals, encourage the use of circular materials or prioritising suppliers who meet rigorous sustainability certifications.

***IN PRACTICE:* EUROPEAN PHASE-OUT LIST (EPOL) FOR CHEMICALS OF CONCERN [4]**

Developed by Health Care Without Harm (HCWH) Europe and leading European healthcare procurement organisations, this common phase-out list of chemicals of concern enables procurement organisations across Europe to select safer alternative products for the healthcare sector.

TIPS FOR SUCCESS

- *Set Clear Sustainability Criteria in Tenders:* Include explicit environmental and social requirements, such as energy efficiency, waste reduction or the use of non-toxic materials, to guide suppliers in developing compliant solutions.
- *Support Pilot Projects:* Encourage suppliers to test and refine their solutions in real-world healthcare settings, offering feedback and paving the way for broader implementation.
- *Use Outcome-Based Specifications:* Focus on the desired results, such as lower environmental impact or improved patient safety, rather than prescribing specific products, allowing suppliers to propose innovative approaches.

> ***IN PRACTICE*: SUSTAINABLE PROCUREMENT CRITERIA – EXAMINATION GLOVES [5]**
>
> HCWH Europe's Plastics Working Group, part of the Healthcare Market Transformation Network, has developed standardised tender criteria to address key sustainability issues in the use of examination gloves within European healthcare. Inspired by Sweden's sustainable procurement criteria for disposable gloves, this resource provides a framework for procurers to align with local policies and sustainability goals, ensuring more sustainable purchasing practices.

COMMON CHALLENGES IN SUSTAINABLE PROCUREMENT OF INNOVATION

Budget Constraints or Perceived Higher Costs

Sustainable products and services often have higher upfront costs compared to traditional options, which can deter organisations operating under tight budgets. Additionally, procurement teams may struggle to demonstrate the long-term value and cost-effectiveness of sustainable choices. This means decision-makers may prioritise short-term savings over long-term sustainability benefits, slowing the adoption of greener practices.

Solution

Focus on lifecycle cost analysis (LCA) to highlight the financial benefits of reduced energy consumption, waste management savings and enhanced durability. Advocate for sustainability as an investment.

> ***BEST PRACTICE:* REDUCING PLASTIC IN HEALTHCARE [6]**
>
> HCWH Europe has created a new resource providing best practice examples of reducing plastic in healthcare. These solutions can support and inspire healthcare facilities to improve circularity by significantly reducing plastics, especially single use. Many of these initiatives can also lead to cost savings. This resource is only available for Global Green and Healthy Hospitals members.

Limited Market Readiness for Sustainable Solutions

The market may not yet offer sustainable solutions that fully meet the organisation's needs or comply with established sustainability criteria. Suppliers might lack the capacity, technology or resources to provide innovative and environmentally friendly products or services. This limits the options available to procurers, potentially forcing them to compromise on sustainability goals or delay procurement initiatives.

Solution

Collaborate with suppliers to co-develop solutions, engage in pre-market consultations and leverage joint procurement efforts to signal demand for sustainable alternatives.

ACTIONABLE TIPS

To effectively incorporate sustainability and innovation into procurement, consider the following actionable tips:

Integrate sustainability into strategy
Ensure sustainability and innovation are embedded in your organisational strategy, with clear objectives and measurable outcomes tied to procurement practices.

Engage leadership and stakeholders

Secure the support of senior leadership and involve key stakeholders early to align priorities and foster a culture that values sustainable innovation.

Leverage collaboration

Work with peers, suppliers and networks to share knowledge, best practices and resources, enabling collective progress toward sustainable solutions.

Adopt long-term thinking

Prioritise long-term value over short-term costs by considering the lifecycle impact of procurement decisions, from production to disposal.

CLOSING REMARKS

Sustainable procurement of innovation is more than just a strategy: it is an opportunity to create real, lasting change. Through our work with Procure4Health, we have been able to demonstrate how procurement can be a powerful tool for driving sustainability in healthcare. In this project our focus has been on collaborating with key stakeholders to identify critical sustainability needs and engage with the market to explore innovative solutions. By aligning our efforts with the right suppliers and understanding market capabilities, we have laid the groundwork for sustainable procurement practices that can transform healthcare systems. Although we have not tested solutions yet, the collaborative approach in Procure4Health has already set the stage for impactful, long-term change. Moving forward, we will continue to build on this foundation, working to bring forward sustainable and innovative solutions that will help shape a healthier, more sustainable future for all.

REFERENCES

1. European Commission. (2020). Public procurement for a better environment: Green Public Procurement (GPP) in the EU. https://ec.europa.eu/environment/gpp/
2. McKinsey & Company. (2021). How companies can achieve significant cost savings with sustainability in procurement. https://www.mckinsey.com/
3. Global Green and Healthy Hospitals. (n.d.). Home. Green Hospitals. https://greenhospitals.org/ [Retrieved January 29, 2025]
4. Health Care Without Harm Europe. (n.d.). *European healthcare's phase-out list of chemicals of concern.* Health Care Without Harm. https://europe.noharm.org/resources/european-healthcares-phase-out-list-chemicals-concern [Retrieved January 29, 2025]
5. Health Care Without Harm Europe. (n.d.). *Sustainable procurement criteria for examination gloves.* Health Care Without Harm. https://europe.noharm.org/resources/sustainable-procurement-criteria-examination-gloves [Retrieved January 29, 2025]
6. Health Care Without Harm Europe. (n.d.). *Reducing plastic in healthcare: Best practice.* Health Care Without Harm. https://europe.noharm.org/news/reducing-plastic-healthcare-best-practice [Retrieved January 29, 2025]

9

The Use of Value-Based Approaches in Innovation Procurement

Hamish Laing

INTRODUCTION

As health systems around the world face the significant challenges of growing demand, complexity and cost of care but constrained human and financial resources, many are turning to Value-Based Healthcare (VBHC) as a way of achieving financial sustainability and improving outcomes for patients and populations within the resources available. The procurement of Medicines, Medical Technologies, Diagnostics and Digital Healthcare is the greatest expenditure for health systems after salaries and wages and so is a critical component of the health ecosystem. It is now recognised that a relentless focus on the lowest price in procurement may not be achieving the best value for patients or their health systems. Consequently, there is increasing interest in Value-Based Procurement (VBP): aligning the reimbursement for goods and services with the outcomes and value they create for patients and the ecosystem. This also emphasises the important role that procurement professionals, working with their clinical colleagues, play in the delivery of great care that meets the needs of patients, is of high quality and measurable.

The public consultation by the European Commission to evaluate the performance of the Public Procurement Directives (2014) specifically requested an assessment in light of current challenges, including resilience considerations and coherence with other EU initiatives [1]. Not only does the consultation open the door to advocating for a shift towards VBP but also helps know how it can be leveraged to support other policy goals, such as the environmental and social responsibility objectives of the EU Supply Chain Directive [2] and the European Green Deal [3], by prioritising sustainable and innovative solutions. The purchasing power of procurement bodies combined with the healthcare decisions that naturally follow from choosing one innovative solution over another makes VBP an extremely influential tool strategically to encourage different stakeholders to engage in the shift towards VBHC.

Whilst VBP can work well for well-established products and services, it is ideally suited to the procurement of innovative technologies, which promise much, but initially may not have an extensive evidence base behind them. However, VBP has requirements that are not present in traditional procurement, and so there is an urgent need to upskill the entire healthcare ecosystem if it is to be successful. This includes policy makers and the managers of the public financing system, procurement professionals, clinicians and suppliers in the technical and cultural changes needed for VBP to be successful and to create shared value for all parties.

Procure4Health VBP Working Group

The importance of VBP as a cross-cutting theme for Innovative Procurement resulted in the creation of a working group of procurement partners in Procure4Health: Danny Havenith of MercurHosp, Belgium; Marco Pantera, Gianluca Carletti, Luminita Costea and Elisa D'Autilia of ARIA, Italy; Harald Johnsen and Ole-Magne Kleven of Sykhusinnkjøp, Norway; Louis Potel of RESAH, France and Carlos Larrañeta Gómez-Caminero from Junta de Andalucia, Spain, supported by Professor Hamish Laing and Dr Helen Yu of the Value-Based Health and Care Academy at Swansea University, Wales, UK.

VALUE-BASED PROCUREMENT OF INNOVATION

Value-Based Procurement (VBP) is a relatively new approach to Innovation Procurement of goods and services that offers procurement professionals the opportunity to support clinical teams to deliver better, measurable outcomes that matter to patients within the resources available. By focusing on getting the best value from the product or service rather than just getting the best price, they can contribute to improved overall system financial sustainability and better patient and population health, which in the medium term will reduce (or at least mitigate the rise) in spending on healthcare. This is aligned to the concepts of personal, technical, allocative and societal value described by the EU Commissions Expert Panel on ways of investing in health in their report about Value-Based Healthcare [4]. Making procurement decisions that are based just on the lowest price is a barrier to the adoption of those innovative technologies which add value through better patient outcomes and improved efficiency.

Value-Based Procurement (sometimes called *Value-Based Pricing*) involves making purchasing decisions that consider how a product or solution can best deliver the outcomes being measured and reduce the total cost of care – rather than focusing exclusively on purchasing a specific product at the lowest possible price[5]. Unlike traditional procurement, VBP typically takes the form of an Outcome-Based Agreement (OBA) where some (usually) or all (rarely) of the payment for the product or service is determined by the achievement of agreed outcome measures. This supports other changes in health system financing that are also being implemented, such as the move away from "fee-for-service" towards "bundled payment" and similar payment models that incentivise allocative and technical value by providers.

This way of engaging with industry suppliers is very different from traditional procurement, which tends to be transactional and sometimes adversarial. It requires a cultural shift for both parties, where the objective is to create shared value from the procurement contract, and makes achieving the outcomes that matter to patients the primary aim. This has been described as a "win-win-win" scenario. In addition, the sharing of risk and reward in these arrangements creates important opportunities to consider the whole pathway of care rather than just the product itself, as it is now in everyone's interest that only patients who will get benefit from the product or intervention are offered it and that it is made available to everyone who will benefit (personal value) at the optimal point in the care pathway (allocative value) and as efficiently as possible (technical value).

VBP differs in other important ways too: instead of the contracting process being concluded once procurement is complete, there needs to be an ongoing relationship with the supplier for the period when outcomes are being captured and measured against the agreed performance, to determine the reimbursement/payment to be made. This also requires data capture, analysis and sharing to "drive" the contract. This reinforces a wider change in the role of procurement departments from the one-off activity of purchasing towards the permanent, high-quality monitoring and measurement of the execution and outcomes of purchasing activities in partnership with the end-users (staff and patients).

One final difference is the need for much closer partnership working between procurement professionals and their health service clients, particularly the senior clinicians. Both groups have significant and specific knowledge and skills which need to be combined for VBP to be successful [6]. This will also be explored further in this Insight.

When thinking about Value-Based Procurement there are several issues to be considered. These can be thought of as Technical and Cultural Success Factors [7].

TECHNICAL SUCCESS FACTORS

What are the practical matters that need to be addressed when undertaking Value-Based Procurement?[8]

When should you use Value-Based Procurement?

It is sometimes argued that there needs to be a strong evidence base for the products or services before VBP can be used. The justification for this is that it "de-risks" the contract for all parties by removing the uncertainty of outcomes that might be achieved. There is no reason why VBP cannot be used in these circumstances, and it allows the outcomes included in the procurement to be more ambitious; however, VBP is ideal for the procurement of new and innovative technologies and services without the usual level of evidence, because VBP allows the risk of achieving the promised outcomes to be shared, for mutual benefit. The patient gains access to the innovation earlier; the supplier can build the evidence base they need for future tenders; and the health system avoids taking all the risk of a relatively unproven innovation, whilst realising the advantages that it promises.

For a VBP to operate effectively, there needs to be an expectation of sufficient use of the procured product or service to generate enough outcomes data and those outcomes must be available and measurable in a timeframe that is appropriate for contracting purposes. This is explored further below.

Which patients or service users does the contract apply to?

Some products or services purchased through VBP will be for all patients with the relevant condition or disease, but that is not always the case. For example, some medicines are licenced for more than one indication and an Outcomes-Based Agreement may only be intended for one of those indications. In Med Tech tenders, there may be various uses of a product:

for instance, for primary vs revisional surgery, and again the VBP may only relate to one use case. It is essential that this is agreed at the outset for two main reasons: firstly, so that the correct data are used to monitor the performance of the product or service over time and thus determine the payment/reimbursement to be made, and secondly, to be able to establish the outcomes baseline for the correct cohort of patients to measure the beneficial change that the product or service creates. The involvement of clinicians in these considerations is essential.

What are the outcomes that will be used?

The primary aim of Value-Based Healthcare and Value-Based Procurement is to improve the outcomes *that matter to the patient (or services user)* at the lowest possible cost, to provide high-value care. There are three distinct groups of outcomes that can be used. The work of ICHOM [9] (ichom.org), who have developed person-centred outcome sets which include CROMs and PROMs, is a useful starting point for many conditions.

Clinical Reported Outcome Measures (CROMs)

Clinical outcomes are typically the most readily available and may have informed the Health Technology Assessment of the innovative technology. Clinical outcomes do matter to patients: for example, survival or good wound healing. However, patients may have many other outcomes that concern them, but which clinicians and the health system do not capture or record. These additional outcomes are best collected by the patient and made available to their clinicians. These are called Patient Reported Outcomes.

Patients Reported Outcomes Measures (PROMs)

These can be added to CROMs to create a more holistic set of outcomes that matter. For example, a patient with cancer is likely to be concerned about their survival (a clinical outcome) but may also want to know if they will get back to doing all the things they enjoyed before they had cancer (measured by PROMs) [10]. A patient undergoing knee replacement surgery will want the implant to last and the wound to heal (clinical outcomes) but may also want to get back to hill running or playing with their grandchildren (PROMs). Patients whose outcome preferences are unlikely to be achieved by a particular treatment may choose less or different intervention.

PROMs are usually developed with patient involvement and scientifically validated by rigorous testing, including in their translation to other languages. PROMs increasingly are being collected from patients using digital platforms compliant with data and interoperability standards to allow capture at scale, repeated over time and shareable. This facilitates their use as part of clinical decision making and potentially for procurement; however, most patients still do not report PROMs for their care across Europe. At the moment, PROMs can only be included in Value-Based Procurement if they are already being captured in the relevant pathway or are introduced alongside the operation of an Outcome-Based Agreement. It is expected that PROMs will become routine in most elective care and long-term conditions as VBHC is implemented across the world and the patient voice is given greater importance by health systems.

Health Resource Utilisation Efficiency ("Technical Value")

Innovation technologies or services will often promise greater efficiency and/or optimisation of the patient pathway as part of their "value proposition". Patients want their care to be efficient as well as to meet their needs and health systems wish to maximise technical value from investments in innovation. VBP is an opportunity to incorporate measures that reflect outcomes of technical value.

Links to Environmental Sustainability

The importance of environmentally sustainable Innovation Procurement has been explored in chapter 8. The connection between environmental sustainability and Value-Based Healthcare is captured by the inclusion of social value, societal value and sustainability as components of any Value-Based Procurement. Firstly, VHBC can lead to reduced demand for interventions and treatment (that would not achieve the outcomes that matter to the patient) and so reduce the environmental impact of health systems. Secondly, Outcome-Based Agreements (OBAs) incentivise health providers and their suppliers to ensure that only patients who are expected to get value from a treatment are offered it. Thirdly, a component of the tender evaluation can specifically relate to environment sustainability measures, such as achieving a reduction in supplier emissions at a corporate or, in time, product level (see figure 9.1).

Where Are the Data and How Will They Be Captured and Shared?

Outcomes used to determine the payment or reimbursement for a product or service need to be:

1. Measurable.
2. Captured as part of routine care or through an additional process.
3. Sufficiently complete.
4. Shareable (with appropriate information governance) with procurement professionals and the supplier.
5. Understood.
6. Comparable with an appropriate baseline.

Careful thought must be given to these factors before an outcome measure is included in a contract. Whilst health data are rarely perfect and can be used despite this, data availability for the outcomes to be included must be established and its level of completeness confirmed. The availability of national or regional registries can be very helpful for this.

Determining who the data controllers ("owners") are and the processes for data sharing must also be agreed, not only between the provider and the team that will operate the contract but also in appropriate form with the supplier, whose income will depend on them. This can take the form of aggregation and pseudonymisation. The use of trusted third parties to manage all the data analysis and reporting is also being explored with blockchain technology and distributed ledgers to allow robust data audit and avoid the need for all the data to be moved into a single database, often from multiple locations with multiple data controllers. Consideration must be given to advising patients of the intended use of their (anonymised) outcomes data for this secondary purpose and obtaining their consent. Expert information governance advice should be obtained. Time spent developing an agreed approach to the use and sharing of data for VBP (with any Data Privacy Impact Assessments and Data Sharing Agreements that are required) will allow subsequent procurements to reuse these principles, avoid duplicating effort and progress more quickly. This could be shared amongst procurement teams as an approach that can be replicated, given that most countries in Europe are operating under the same or similar Data Protection Regulation.

Figure 9.1 Proposed for MedTech in NHS England (2025) (under consultation) [11]

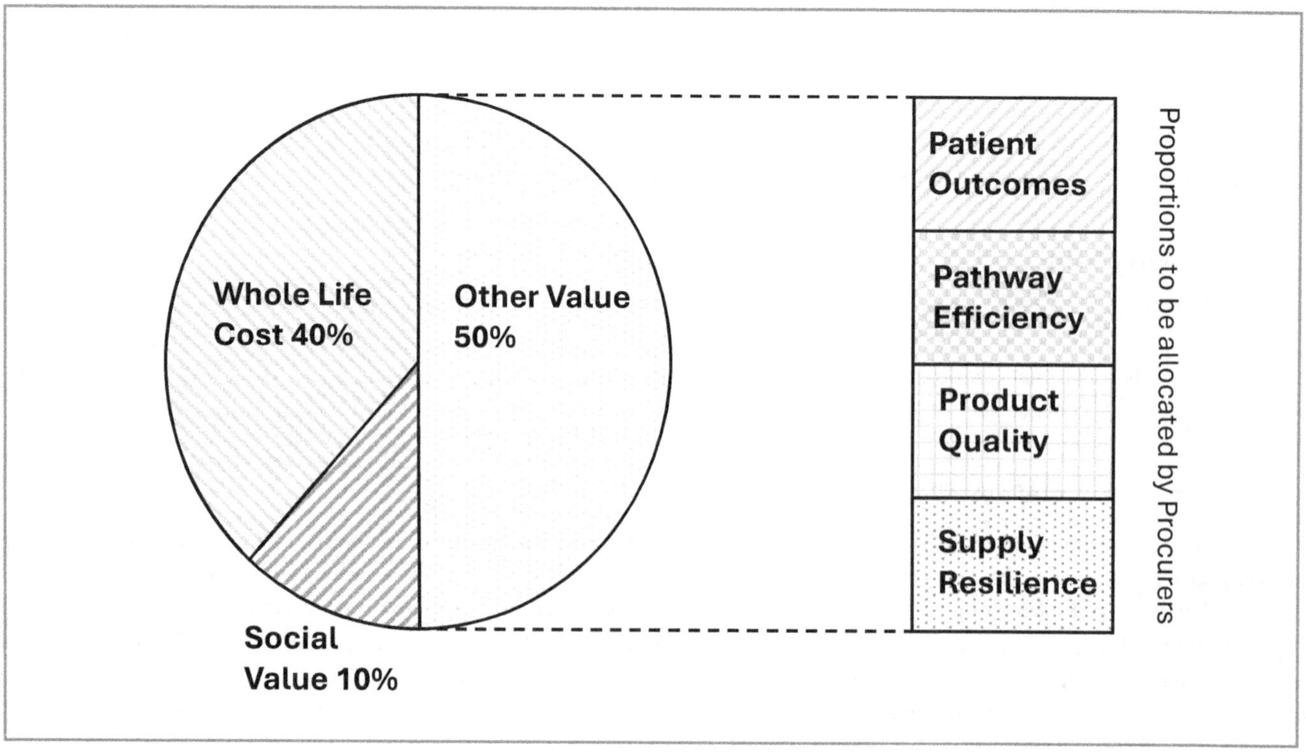

What Is the Design of the Contract?

An important principle for early resolution is whether the contract is a *malus* or *bonus* contract design. Whilst it is most common for a supplier to receive 100% of the cost initially with the requirement for them to make a rebate if the outcomes are not met, this provides little incentive to suppliers to create innovations that achieve better and better outcomes and requires diligent monitoring of contract performance will effective communication between clinical teams (who know the outcomes) and financial teams who must claim the rebate. Bonus contracts where additional reimbursement can occur if outcomes exceed expectations are more aligned with the principle of VBHC and can be capped by design to manage the level of financial risk for providers.

There is also a need to determine how multiple outcomes will be used and which are binary outcomes, and which are linear/graduated outcomes with thresholds. There are advantages and disadvantages of single versus a basket of outcome measures and expert advice may be helpful in choosing the best approach for a particular situation.

Dealing with Clinical Pathway Change

The introduction of innovation can result in significant changes to clinical pathways of care, not all of which can be anticipated. In addition, other factors can impact on how care is delivered or the effectiveness of an innovative technology. This can result in unexpected or perverse outcomes that could not be foreseen when the innovation was procured. It is important to "build in" sufficient flexibility into any Outcomes-Based Agreement to be able to review and adapt the measures and performance requirements in such circumstances. Including contract review points into the agreement can be helpful in this respect.

CULTURAL SUCCESS FACTORS

Value-Based Procurement requires both technical and cultural change in how procurement teams, provider clinicians and suppliers interact. It is important that trust is built between suppliers and their customers to facilitate the success of this very different way of procuring innovation and is akin to a longer-term partnership to solve problems facing clinical teams rather than a short term, transactional interaction to purchase a product. Smaller scale OBAs with relatively few outcomes can help develop experience and trust between parties as the basis for larger scale and more ambitious VBPs in the future.

Pathway Thinking

VBP is an opportunity to think more broadly across the whole clinical pathway and about how greater (and shared) value can be released by the introduction of innovation. Does the innovation allow steps in the pathway to be removed or resources allocated differently? Using the innovation to review and reduce cost in a pathway can greatly increase the value of an intervention even if the outcomes remain unchanged. This approach can expose and reduce unwarranted variation in how care is provided. Can the supplier support the management of the service change or pathway redesign as "added value" in the contract? With payment/reimbursement dependent in part on outcomes, there are incentives to ensure the only right patients are getting the innovative intervention at the right time, but also that every patient who may get value from that innovation is offered it.

Working with Clinicians

VBP cannot succeed without a closer partnership between procurement professionals and clinical leaders. Clinicians can help identify the procurement need, define the patient "cohorts" to be included, help agree (with patient advocates) the outcomes to be measured and the baseline, and assist with the interpretation of the outcomes data that result. It is rare for clinicians to have a good understanding of procurement regulations or processes and so the combination of procurement professionals and clinicians is essential to ensure success and with time can become increasingly effective. Learning about VBP together can help to build relationships between these two professional groups.

Supplier Readiness

There has been a great focus on the requirements of procurement teams and healthcare providers to implement Value-Based Procurement of innovation but there is also a need for life sciences companies to work differently if they are to engage appropriately and successfully in such tenders. This requires the supplier to be "internally ready" for VBHC, not just in their customer facing teams (market access, sales) but across the whole business (c-suite, finance, legal, marketing, government affairs, etc.) and to have innovative business models and internal incentives available that are aligned with VBHC: a concept we have described as *Value-Based Supply* [12–13]. Procurers may wish to assure themselves that potential suppliers have sufficient Value-Based Supply maturity to be included in any Value-Based Procurement.

Education and Training

As with every business change, the introduction of Value-Based Procurement for innovation requires new knowledge and skills. Lack of the relevant knowledge amongst the procurement profession specifically, and the ecosystem more generally, about how to design and operate VBP in practice has been identified as a barrier to adoption. This means educational programmes with a focus on the practicalities will be critically important and there is merit is some joint education between clinicians, procurement professionals as well as industry suppliers. It is also vital that there is open and shared learning between procurement teams about what works and what doesn't and why. A community of practice approach for procurement professionals could be very helpful with this and the provision of ongoing education.

NEXT STEPS FOR VALUE-BASED PROCUREMENT OF INNOVATION

Procurement Teams

For procurement teams to implement Value-Based Procurement successfully into their business there are some key steps that should be followed:

- **Secure executive management support:**
  - Ensure directors, general managers and senior clinical colleagues understand and endorse the principles of VBP. Engage them in developing value-based tenders and monitoring contract performance.
- **Take stock, internally and externally:**
  - Assess the readiness of your procurement team and healthcare provider. Invest in training and education and share knowledge and good practice.
- **Check if suppliers are ready for VBP:**
  - Ensure that suppliers are internally ready (Value-Based Supply) and prepared to work with VBP. Learn from those already applying VBP in other markets.
- **Decide when to use VBP:**
  - VBP may not always be appropriate. Start with simple tenders where outcome data are measurable and available.
- **Understand the process and tools required to create an Outcomes-Based Agreement:**
  - Engage with clinical and patient organisations, select outcomes, collect data, design the contract and manage the incentives and financials.
- **Evaluate and share learning:**
  - Report on value-based approaches and share lessons with the procurement community.

Healthcare Providers

In addition, there are some essential structural conditions that must be met within the healthcare provider:

- There must be a structured approach to innovation, ideally with a Chief Innovation Officer at C-level. This person is responsible for working with clinicians and patient representatives to identify needs and for communication between the individual stakeholders, which include clinicians, procurement teams, suppliers and academia.
- There should be a project approach that integrates innovative projects into existing organisational structures efficiently and adopts the principles of Impactful Innovation to anticipate and avoid adoption failure.

- Internal and external communication amongst all stakeholders in innovative procurement is vital. It should be open and transparent and should include patients and their representatives. This is critical to build trust in the approach, maintain engagement as well as to disseminate learning.
- Such is the strategic and financial importance of procurement for providers, inclusion of a senior procurement professional within the provider leadership team will ensure co-ordination of procurement activities across the clinical, finance and innovation portfolios and thus maximise the likelihood of benefits realisation and appropriate prioritisation. It will also support earlier procurement involvement in innovation investment decisions and importantly identify opportunities for Value-Based Procurement at an early stage.

CLOSING REMARKS

Value-Based Procurement is not only well suited to Innovation Procurement but is fully aligned with the adoption of Value-Based Healthcare by health systems wanting to deliver high value care with better outcomes within the resources available to them, and to reduce healthcare expenditure over the medium- to long-term. VBP is an important part of creating economically and environmentally sustainable health systems in the face of increasingly challenging circumstances and helps avoids the purchase of lower cost products and services which ultimately prove to be of low value and a poor investment.

VBP allows shared value to be achieved by all parties: patients, providers and suppliers and supports the introduction of innovations that benefits patients earlier than might otherwise be the case. It is also a key driver to reducing low value care and incentivising higher value interventions through innovation putting procurement teams at the heart of the achievement of better health outcomes.

VBP is a new and different way of working for procurement professionals, their provider customers, clinicians and life sciences industry suppliers. Initially it will be more resource intensive and complicated, and it will take time for procurement professionals and suppliers to become skilled and confident in the approach. This "learning curve" can be shortened by high-quality educational programmes, research and evaluation of completed Value-Based Procurements. A willingness to share learning within the procurement community about what worked, what did not, and the reasons for that is essential. All of this will build trust within the ecosystem and allow initial small-scale and less complex Value-Based Procurements to be expanded to larger scale and ambition, ensuring that the greatest value is achieved through the procurement process, whilst incentivising industry to continue innovate to meet the needs of patients and the challenges of modern healthcare.

REFERENCES

1. https://single-market-economy.ec.europa.eu/news/commission-launches-call-evidence-and-public-consultation-evaluation-public-procurement-directives-2024-12-13_en (Accessed 23 April 2025).
2. https://commission.europa.eu/business-economy-euro/doing-business-eu/sustainability-due-diligence-responsible-business/corporate-sustainability-due-diligence_en (Accessed 23 April 2025).
3. https://commission.europa.eu/strategy-and-policy/priorities-2019-2024/european-green-deal_en (Accessed 23 April 2025).
4. Expert Panel on effective ways of investing in Health (EXPH). (26 June 2019). Defining Value in "Value-based Healthcare". https://health.ec.europa.eu/publications/defining-value-value-based-healthcare_en (Accessed 1 March 2025).
5. Steele R, Paardekooper C, Steenhuis S and Boonen L. (December 2022). Talking Value: A Taxonomy on Value-Based Healthcare. EU Alliance for Value in Health. https://www.europeanallianceforvalueinhealth.eu/library/talking-value-a-taxonomy-on-value-based-healthcare/ (Accessed 20 March 2025).
6. Matinheikki J, Kenny K, Kauppi K, van Raaij E and Brandon-Jones A. (2024). Realising the Promise of Value-based Purchasing: Experimental Evidence of Medical Device Selection. *International Journal of Operations & Production Management*, Vol. 44 No. 13, pp. 100–126. https://doi.org/10.1108/IJOPM-09-2023-0779.
7. Bohm N, Bermingham S, Grimsey Jones F, Goncalves-Bradley DC, Diamantopoulos A. Burton JR and Laing H. (2021). The Challenges of Outcomes-Based Contract Implementation for Medicines in Europe. *PharmacoEconomics.* https://doi.org/10.1007/s40273-021-01070-1.
8. Burton JR, Halsby K, Sáinz de la Fuente G, Pearson-Stuttard J et al. (2024). Value-Based Healthcare in Practice: IDEATE, a Collaboration to Design and Test an Outcomes-Based Agreement for a Medicine in Wales. *PharmacoEconomics.* https://doi.org/10.1007/s40273-024-01445-0.

9. Sets of Patient-Centered Outcome Measures. https://www.ichom.org/patient-centered-outcome-measures/ (Accessed 10 April 2025).
10. Cole A, Cubi-Molla P, Pollard J, Sim D, Sullivan R, Sussex J and Lorgelly P. (2019). Making Outcome-Based Payment a Reality in the NHS. http://www.cancerresearchuk.org.
11. https://www.nhsprocurement.org.uk/news/Help-to-shape-a-new-evaluation-methodology-for-Value-Based-Procurement-of-medical-technology (Accessed 14 April 2025).
12. Laing H and McHale J. Value-Based Supply: Re-imagining Value from Within. https://www.europeanallianceforvalueinhealth.eu/publication/value-based-supply-re-imagining-value-from-within/ (Accessed 30 March 2025).
13. Laing H, Yu, H, Rich N and McHale J. Value-Based Supply: Developing Internal Readiness. https://www.europeanallianceforvalueinhealth.eu/publication/value-based-supply-developing-internal-readiness/ (Accessed 30 March 2025).

FURTHER READING

Bates DW, Deerberg-Wittram J, Katz G, Braeger K et al. (2023). Using Publicly Reported Global Hospital Rankings to Improve Dissemination of Patient-Reported Outcome Measures (PROMs). *NEJM Catal Innov Care Deliv*, Vol. 4 No. 11. htpps://doi.org/10.1056/CAT.23.0097.

Gerecke G, Clawson J, Pross C, Verboven Y and Bax H. (2020). How Procurement Unlocks Value-Based Health Care. Boston Consulting Group. https://www.bcg.com/publications/2020/procurement-unlocks-value-based-health-care.

Pedroso CB, Beaulieu M, Allerup LD and Rebolledo C. (January 2022). Fostering Innovation through Procurement in the Healthcare Sector: The Danish Experience. *Healthc Q*. Vol. 24 No. 4, pp. 22–26. htpps://doi.org/10.12927/hcq.2022.26715.

Index

Page numbers in *italics* indicate figures and tables.